HERBAL
FIRST AID
and
HEALTH CARE

Medicine for a
New Millennium

KYLE D. CHRISTENSEN, D.C., M.H.

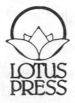

Published by:
Lotus Press
P.O. Box 325, Twin Lakes, Wisconsin 53181 USA

DISCLAIMER

This guide to not meant to represent definitive guidelines for the treatment of illness or injury. As with any injury or health concern competent professional treatment is recommended. For goodness sake, use your common sense.

COVER & PAGE DESIGN/LAYOUT: Paul Bond, Art & Soul Design
ILLUSTRATIONS: Curtis Wiens
AUTHOR PHOTO: Annita Stenken

First Edition, 2000

Printed in the United States of America

Herbal First Aid & Health Care, Medicine for a New Millenium includes bibliographical references.
ISBN 0-914955-90-X
Library of Congress Control Number 99-96594

Published by:
Lotus Press, P.O. Box 325, Twin Lakes, Wisconsin 53181
web: www.lotuspress.com
e-mail: lotuspress@lotuspress.com
800-824-6396

DEDICATION

To my children and to yours.

To my eternal partner and wife, Trish, whose sacrifice,
support and devotion to myself and our children
make life the worthwile adventure that it is.

ACKNOWLEDGMENTS

Randy Giboney -
my partner in herbs and our company, Western Botanicals.
When we first met, he ran my first marathon with me to
support me and has been running with me ever since
(figuratively and literally). A better friend cannot be found.

Tim Jackson, D.C. -
a friend and partner in the healing arts. Thanks for
your willingness to completely tear up a manuscript
or article and give positive feedback.

Steve Tristant, D.P.M. -
for his example in patient care and management and his
ability to discuss and explain things with his patients.

Christian Pebbles, E.M.T. -
for his skill and enthusiasm as a
fireman and emergency medical technician.

Kaleem Joy -
Certified Nurse Midwife for her devotion
and dedication to the art of midwifery.

Curtis Wiens -
whose computer and graphics expertise took
the worry of illustrations away from me.

TABLE OF CONTENTS

Chapter 12 - Bites & Stings 183

Chapter 13 - Mouth & Dental Problems 191

PREFACE

The concepts and practices taught in this volume are presented as educational material which can be used in case of emergency when help is on the way as well as when no immediate help is available. This book contains many unconventional practices and concepts. The application of the educational material contained herein may cause adverse reactions in some people. Many ideas contained in this volume are not medically proven and are considered by some to be unorthodox. Before following any of these unproven ideas, please consult with your own medical doctor. Contrary to the belief of some, herbs can cause adverse or allergic reactions in some people.

The opinions expressed in this document are those of the author and are for educational purposes only. If you feel you must self medicate, do so with extreme caution. Do not endanger yourself. When conditions are misdiagnosed or treated incorrectly, natural and herbal methods can be as harmful as any other treatment.

The publisher and the author of this book assumes no responsibility for the correct or incorrect use of this information. No treatment should be rendered without the express approval and guidance of your family doctor. The information in this book is designed to increase public awareness of various types of injuries and/or illnesses and herbal and natural therapies that have been used in the past for such conditions.

Any natural method of treatment can backfire and harm an individual, particularly if the condition is misdiagnosed or not understood. This is why it is important to call for assistance (CALL 911) or consult with your family physician. This book is not designed to replace competent medical care. Overzealousness and a disdain for the current politics of the medical system is no excuse to exercise poor judgment or reckless practices, particularly when a life is at stake. All are admonished to use good common sense, recognize your limitations (and lack of training) and call for help when necessary.

- *Kyle D. Christensen, D.C., M.H.*
January 1999

INTRODUCTION

In the field of natural healing, modern emergency medicine is unsurpassed in its lifesaving techniques and ancient herbal wisdom should be the treatment of choice for chronic or degenerative conditions. However, as this text will reveal, herbs can have an important part in the treatment of emergency situations. Too often the uninformed view herbal medicine as sipping savory teas to settle an upset tummy. While herbal teas are highly visible, the full spectrum of herbal medicines can also initiate dramatic physiologic responses that can and do save lives. As many medical dogmas and beliefs are beginning to fall into disfavor, the benefits of natural healthcare are enjoying a renaissance. Herbal traditions have been passed down from one generation to the next for one simple reason. They work. In fact, the plant kingdom is responsible for the basis of most of modern pharmacology. By staying within "Mother Nature's" original versions of medicines, modern researchers are finding very favorable results without the oppressive side effects.

Many of the most useful first aid books, that go into any depth, require a first aid pharmacy that only a licensed medical doctor or pharmacist could have access to. Which would be okay if you practiced medicine, but most of us do not. Nor do we want to. The strength of HERBAL FIRST AID, is that not only does it work, but it is also available to each of us. And even if drugs are unavailable to you, as long as you have the earth, sun and water, you can have your herbal medicines.

We do not have to go back too many generations to find that our grandparents and great grandparents were very closely tied to the earth. Many of us are once again feeling a kinship with the earth. Science is validating what the ancients have taught us all along. Herbal treatment or medicine should not be construed as inferior when compared to using chemical or synthetic drugs. When properly administered, herbs can be just as effective and often more effective than their pharmaceutical counterparts.

You will note a certain amount of redundancy in many of the herbal recommendations or treatment protocols. It is not because we are limited with herbal resources, rather it is to emphasize the principles involved in natural healing. Namely, cleansing the body of toxins and impurities and nourishing and assisting the body in rebuilding and healing. There are thousands of herbs that are used medicinally in the world, yet it is not necessary to know and use even 100. If you were to thoroughly use and understand only 10 medicinal herbs you would not be lacking because herbs are multi-faceted in their uses. Which means that the same herb can help many different conditions. **This books emphasis is to help you to identify the nature of the conditions you may encounter, then teach you appropriate ways to respond.**

Herbal therapies can be both safe and effective. Of course, it is important that you also learn when you are over your head and need help. We must not only learn, but exercise good judgment. It will not always be your call to be an "Herbal Hero".

When injuries or sudden illness occurs, there is a critical period of time in which taking action is of the utmost importance to the outcome of the situation. What you do, or what you don't do, during this time may mean the difference between a quick resolution of symptoms or even life and death. You owe it to yourself, your family, friends and neighbors to know and to understand procedures that you can apply quickly and effectively in an emergency. The Boy Scouts of America have a motto, "Be Prepared". The time for preparation is now. Learn the lifesaving skills and herbal wisdom taught in this book. Begin with your own herbal medicine garden, growing medicinal herbs that will not only beautify your home, but provide you with vital and potentially lifesaving herbs.

By combining the benefits of medical lifesaving knowledge and herbal wisdom, you are able to provide the most effective and immediate care or "First Aid".

Read the material contained in this book carefully. Practice the techniques with family and friends before an emergency arises. **Enroll in a Red Cross First Aid and CPR course.** Keep this book in your Herbal First Aid Kit or where it will be on hand for quick reference when needed.

- Kyle D. Christensen, D.C., N.D., M.H.

FIRST THINGS FIRST

The key to helping someone who has become ill or injured is to go about their treatment in a logical methodical manner so that you are able to quickly assess and stabilize the condition.

If you follow an organized procedure, you will not overlook problems that may not be obvious.

Begin with your ABC's as part of your PRIMARY SURVEY then on to a more detailed examination in the SECONDARY SURVEY.

PRIMARY SURVEY

Survey the scene

Before you tend to the person, assess the scene. Accidents tend to multiply. Make sure that everything is safe for the rescuers and the victim before you begin treatment. Look for any immediate hazard that may result in more injuries. If you jump into the scene prematurely, you may become part of the problem and will need help yourself.

THE A,B,C'S:

Airway

If the person can talk, then the airway is functioning and they are able to breathe. With an unconscious person, place your ear next to their nose and mouth and put your hand on their chest. Look, listen and feel for movement (the chest raising and lowering). If the person is unconscious and their head is down or in a position that may not allow for open breathing, you must gently move the head to open the airway.

If there is no air movement, check to see if the tongue is blocking the airway by pushing down on the forehead while lifting the chin. If you suspect a possible neck injury, you can open the airway by lifting the jaw without moving the neck.

If there is still no air movement, pinch the persons' nose and seal your mouth over theirs and try to force air into their lungs. If the chest does not rise, there is probably an obstruction. Perform the Heimlich maneuver to open the airway (see page 27).

Perform Artificial Respiration until the person can breath on their own (see page 18).

Breathing

Make sure the person is breathing. Look for the rise and fall of the chest. Feel the breath from the mouth or under the nose. If the person is not breathing, check for their pulse to determine whether you should perform just artificial respiration or CPR.

Circulation

Check for circulation by placing your index and middle fingertips into the hollow of the neck below the angle of the person's jaw feeling for the carotid pulse. If there is no pulse begin CPR (see page 24). If the pulse is slow, weak or irregular make a mental note and re-check in a few minutes.

Severe Bleeding

Check quickly for severe blood loss or bleeding. Check both visually and with your hands. Slide your hands under the patient and within bulky clothing for hidden blood loss or bleeding. Control bleeding by direct pressure, administration of cayenne pepper (tincture orally, powder externally), elevating the injured site (if reasonable), direct pressure on a pressure point or the use of a tourniquet.

Cervical Spine (The Neck)

During your primary survey of the person, be careful to keep the neck and head as still as possible if you suspect there could be any injury to the neck (cervical spine). If the person is unconscious, has fallen from a height, experienced an blow to the head or a sudden acceleration or deceleration (such as in an auto accident) you should be suspicious. See treatment of cervical spine injuries page 77.

If the person does have a possible spinal cord injury, you still may need to move the patient to safety. (see Moving an Injured Person, page 37). To move the person, grasp the sides of the person's head firmly and gently traction the neck attempting to align the head with the rest of the body. Gentle traction should be maintained until mechanical traction can be made or improvised (see neck injury, page 76).

SECONDARY SURVEY

The Physical Exam

When the immediate threats to life have been controlled, you must systematically inspect the entire person, evaluating the extent of the known injuries and look for any unsuspected pain or bodily damages. Depending on the situation your exam will be more or less thorough.

General guidelines for the person examination include:

1. Gently but firmly palpate (feel) all relevant body parts, looking for obvious damage, pain responses, swelling, deformities, and abnormalities. If the person can talk ask them where it hurts, or feels bad.

2. Move the patient as little as possible and avoid aggravating any known injuries.

3. When necessary cut away any clothing to visualize any suspected injuries. It is best to cut clothes away rather than risk further injury by removing the clothes in a way that bends the arms, legs or spinal cord. (Except if the clothes are new or your favorite - *just kidding*)

4. Talk with the patient through the entire process, even if they appear unconscious. This will comfort and keep the patient informed, which is psychologically very important.

Begin at the head of the person "LAF-ing all the way" (LAF = looking, asking, feeling). You are seeking for signs and symptoms of the problems. Systematically examine the person quite literally from head to toe.

HEAD: Look for damage, discoloration, and blood or fluid draining from the ears, nose, and mouth. Ask about loss of consciousness, pain, or any abnormal sensations. Feel for lumps, dents and deformities.

NECK: Look for obvious damage, and make sure the trachea (throat) is lined up in the midline of the neck. Feel along the sides and back of the neck (the cervical spine) for any pain.

SHOULDERS AND ARMS: One at a time, squeeze each shoulder, and run down the arms to the fingers. Check for increased or poor circulation (one arm or hand feels hotter or colder to you). Check sensation and motion of fingers. Pinch the finger tips to check for capillary refilling. Look at the fingernails to see how fast blood returns. Compare to the other hand if necessary.

CHEST: Gently but firmly press down on the sternum (breast bone). Compress the ribs from both sides, keeping your hands wide to prevent the possibility of too much direct pressure on fractures. This will find a rib fracture very quickly. Look for damage or deformities. Ask about pain. Feel for any instability. Have the patient take in a deep breath and monitor for pain.

ABDOMEN: With hands apart, press gently on the abdomen in each of the four quadrants (right upper, left upper, right lower, left lower). Make a note of which quadrant(s) were painful. Look for any damage. Ask about pain and discomfort. Feel for rigidity, distention, or muscle spasms.

BACK: Look at the back if possible for signs of trauma or deformity. Slide your hands under the patient, palpating as much of the spine as possible feeling for areas of pain, muscle spasm or swelling.

PELVIS: Cup the iliac crests with your hands (the hip bones at your waist), pressing gently down, and squeezing toward the midline of the body. Ask about pain. Feel for instability.

LEGS: With your hands surrounding each leg, one at a time, run from the groin down to the toes, squeezing as you go. Look for any swelling, pain, or deformities. Check the circulation, sensations and motion of toes.

A written or dictated note of all the possible injuries should be kept. Take the time to do a thorough exam even though you think you may know the extent of the injuries.

VITAL SIGNS: Vital signs are used to let you know how the person is doing. Become aware of what the normal is and you will be better able to assess the person. These include breathing, pulse rate, blood pressure, etc. . .

LEVEL OF CONSCIOUSNESS: A person with a normal level of consciousness will be able to communicate with you. They will know their name, where they are, and generally what time it is. The level of consciousness is the easiest sign to assess and the first to change. Consciousness can be graded using the AVPU scale ranging from alert to unresponsive.

Alert: The person seems normal, and answers intelligently about person, place and time. They know essentially what happened to them.

Verbal: The person is not alert, but they do respond in some way when spoken to.

Pain: The person does not react to verbal stimuli, but they do react to pain, being pinched or rubbed in sensitive areas.

Unresponsive: The person does not respond to stimuli.

PULSE: In your primary assessment you noted the pulse at the carotid artery. This lets you know that blood is being pumped from the heart to the brain. Next pay attention to the rate, rhythm and quality of the pulse. Use the radial pulse found on the inside of the wrist below the thumb. Press lightly with your index and middle fingers.

Rate: This means the number of beats per minute. A range of 60-80 is normal for an adult. It is usually higher in children, sometimes reaching 160 beats per minutes in an infant. Counting for one full minute is the most accurate, but counting for 15 seconds and multiplying by 4 is the most commonly used. If you don't have a watch, check the pulse anyway for the rhythm and quality.

Rhythm: There will be either a clock-like regularity, or a sporadic irregularity.

Quality: This refers to the force exerted by the heart on each beat. A normal quality is strong. A "thready" pulse is weak and an indication of inadequate circulation, and a "bounding" pulse is abnormally forceful.

If you cannot find a radial pulse check the other arm. An absence on one side could mean an injury to the arm or shoulder. A weak pulse could be an indication that the person could be going into shock.

Increasing pulse rate, see shock, page 39

Deformed fracture causing decreased pulse, see page 72-74

RESPIRATION: Do not let the patient know you are checking their respiration because often they will become self conscious and alter their breathing pattern.

Rate: An adult normally breathes 12-18 times per minute. Children and infants breath faster.

Rhythm: Normally, we breathe evenly and regularly, exhalations taking slightly longer than inhalations. Watch for shallowness or deepness, and irregularities in the pattern.

Quality: Normal breathing is quiet and effortless. Abnormal breathing might include labor, pain, noise (snores, squeaks, gurgles, gasps), and a flaring of the nostrils.

SKIN: It keeps the outside out and the insides in. The skin breathes, filters and protects the body's core. The skin gives pertinent information on the general well-being of the patient.

Color: Pink is the normal color of skin in the non-pigmented areas (the lining of the eyes, inside the mouth, fingernail beds. It may be difficult to detect subtle changes in skin color with darker complexions. The size of the blood vessels near the skin determine the color. Vasodilatation (widening of blood vessels) produces a red, flushed color, and indicates problems such as fever or hypothermia. Vasoconstriction (narrowing of blood vessels) produces pale or blotchy skin, and may be an indication of shock or hypothermia. A blue hue, called cyanosis, indicates a lack of oxygen, such as in heart failure or gas poisoning. Yellowish skin can indicate liver failure or disease.

Fever, see page 166

Shock, see page 39

Hypothermia, see page 154

Yellow skin, see jaundice, page 168

Temperature: The temperature of the skin can be significantly lower than the body's core and still be perfectly healthy. It will indicate, though, whether the person is vasodilating and growing warmer, or vasoconstriction and getting cooler.

Moisture: Normal skin is relatively dry. Warmth and wetness from excessive sweating may be evident, but if the skin is cool and moist, it may indicate shock.

BLOOD PRESSURE: Blood pressure is impossible to take without a device called a sphygmomanometer (blood pressure cuff) and a stethoscope. In most first aid situations, you will not be able to take a person's blood pressure. However, for educational purposes or if you have the proper equipment to take the blood pressure, this is what is going on.

As your heart beats (contracts) blood is pushed out of the heart into the blood vessels. The force of the blood creates pressure against the walls of the arteries and veins. The pressure within the circulatory system is necessary for the oxygen and carbon dioxide transfer to take place on a cellular level. When the blood pressure drops too low for oxygen to be transferred to the tissues, they begin to die. Blood pressure has two components: 1) the systolic pressure, which is the amount of pressure when the heart contracts and a gush or surge of blood is pushing against the arteries, and 2) the diastolic pressure, which measures the resting pressure against the blood vessels in between contractions of the heart. A general normal blood pressure is written as 120/80 (systolic/diastolic). However healthy normal blood pressure varies greatly from person to person. If you have a blood pressure cuff but because of background noise you cannot hear well. You can determine the systolic pressure by palpating the radial pulse at the wrist. The first pulse you will feel as the cuff exhales will be the systolic pressure.

As the blood pressure drops, the skin becomes more and more cyanotic (blue). The pulses begin to disappear. First you lose the pulse in the feet, then your wrists, and finally the neck. If you found a radial (wrist) pulse earlier, but can no longer find it, they are losing pressure. Prior to the blood pressure dropping, the heart attempts to compensate by increasing the pulse rate. If the pulse rate is increasing, try to correct the underlying cause.

Anxiety, see page 205

Fainting, see page 31

Severe allergic reaction/anaphylaxis, see page 93

Blood loss (internal or external), see page 14

MEDICAL HISTORY

Eighty percent of your diagnosis or conclusions will come from the information gathered as you interview the person. Approach the person with a calm, confident attitude, whether you feel like it or not. An aura of calmness surrounding the scene will often do more for the sick and injured than all the splints and herbs you can throw at them. Quietly tell them your name and that you can help them. Don't scream, "What happened, What happened? Or How Stupid! Why did you do that?".

If you haven't already established a relationship with the person. It is more effective to say sincerely, "I know you must be afraid and in pain but we'll make you as comfortable as possible," as opposed to panting, "You'll be OK, you'll be fine."

Be positive about the situation. Ask how you can make them more comfortable. Be honest without saying everything you're thinking. Beware of the tone of your voice. Discuss with them the possible plans of action. They have a right to their say in what happens.

There are several mnemonics that are helpful in taking a medical history.

Ample

ALLERGIES: "Are you allergic to anything you know of?"

MEDICATIONS: "Taking any drugs or medications currently?"

PAST HISTORY: "Has anything like this happened before?" Is there anything I should know about your health?"

LAST MEAL: "When did you eat or drink last?"

EVENTS: "What led up to this?", and "Is there anything else I should know?"

A mnemonic for assessing pain or discomfort if PQRST. Ask them to describe the pain for you.

What **PROVOKES** the pain?

What is the **QUALITY** of the pain?

Does it **RADIATE**?

Describe the **SEVERITY**

What **TIME** did it start?

If the patient is unconscious check and see if they are wearing a Medical Alert tag on their neck, wrist or ankles. Check pockets for information. Ask witnesses. Seek answers to the A-E-I-O-U TIPS. Is their unconsciousness due to ALLERGIES, EPILEPSY, INFECTION, OVERDOSE, UNDER-DOSE, TRAUMA, INSULIN, PSYCHOLOGICAL disorder, or STROKE?

SOAP NOTES

If time allows or there are others at the scene, record the information from your assessment. You will not remember everything unless it is written down. Your notes can be divided into four sections

SUBJECTIVE: What happened to who (include age, address, and sex), where, and when? What is the chief complaint?

OBJECTIVE: What did the physical exam reveal? What are the vital signs and when did you do the following checks? What is the relevant medical history?

ASSESSMENT: What are the possible problems?

PLAN: What are you going to do?

Add to the notes your name and the names of any other members of the aiding party and witnesses.

Repeat your SOAP notes with each reassessment, which may need to be every 15 minutes in very serious situations or after a couple of hours for less urgent situations.

REVIEW OF ASSESSMENT & STABILIZATION

First Things First

1. Stay calm and think first before you act.

2. CALL 911, or have someone else CALL 911. If there is a crisis or true emergency, now is not the time to be an "herbal hero to the rescue". Our society has trained very skilled and competent professionals that have handled more emergencies than most of us ever will.

3. When you approach an injured person, think of the ABC's:

   A = Airway. Make sure the victims airway is not blocked by the tongue, secretions or some foreign body (see page 18 - artificial respiration, and choking - page 27)

   B = Breathing. Make sure the person is breathing. If not administer artificial respiration (page 18)

   C = Circulation. Make sure the patient has a pulse. If no pulse is felt, administer CPR (cardiopulmonary resuscitation) (see page 24)

4. Check for severe bleeding.

5. Act fast if the victim is bleeding severely(see page 14), or if he has swallowed poison (see page 157), or if his heart or breathing has stopped. Every second counts.

6. Although most injured persons can be safely moved, it is vitally important not to move a person with a serious neck or back injury - unless you have to save him from further danger (see pages 76, 37 [neck/back injuries, moving an injured person])

7. Keep the person lying down and quiet. If he has vomited- and there is no danger that his neck is broken (see page 76) - turn him on his side to prevent choking. Examine for shock. (Shock is a serious condition of acute circulatory collapse, usually brought on by severe blood loss or trauma).

8. Begin treating the person accordingly using a good "bedside manner", calming and reassuring the person to help prevent shock or hysteria.

9. Find adequate shelter for the injured person, out of the harsh elements. Keep the person warm, calm and reassured that all is going well.

10. Have someone call for medical assistance while you apply first aid. The person who calls for help should be able to explain the nature of the emergency and ask what should be done pending the arrival of the ambulance.

11. Examine the victim gently. Cut the clothing, if necessary, to avoid abrupt movement or added pain. Don't pull clothing away from burns unless it's still smoldering (see page 22)

12. Don't give fluids to an unconscious or semiconscious person; fluids may enter his windpipe and cause suffocation. Don't try to arouse an unconscious person by slapping or shaking.

13. Look for an emergency medical identification card or emblematic device that the victim may be wearing to alert you to any health problems- allergies or diseases that require special care.

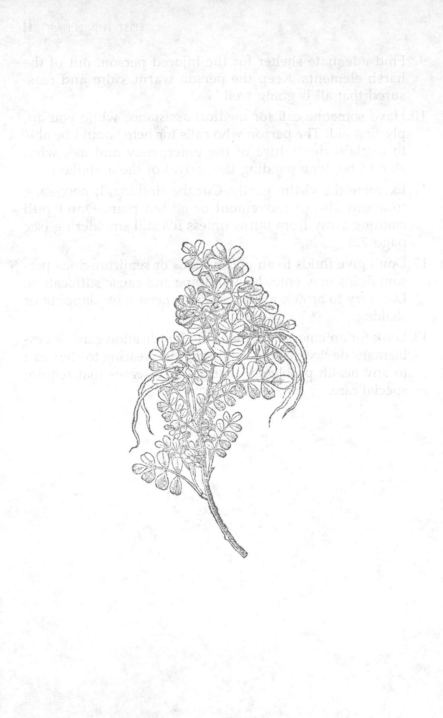

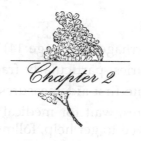

Chapter 2

LIFE THREATENING EMERGENCIES

AUTOMOBILE ACCIDENTS

Nothing is likely to test one's knowledge of first aid more than an accident on the highway. Injuries may be severe; you may be a great distance from professional help. Keep a copy of this Handbook in your car, along with a first-aid kit. In addition keep the following supplies in your car:

- Blanket to keep an injured person covered and to move him (see page 37)
- Warning lights or flares to be used if car is stalled.

In giving first aid, remember that moving the victim, making a hasty attempt to get him out of the car, may do untold harm, particularly if there are arm or leg fractures or spinal injuries are involved.

Give first aid at once, inside the vehicle whenever possible, before attempting to move the injured person. Exceptions: 1- when the vehicle is on fire; 2- when gasoline has been spilled and fire hazard is great; 3- when you are in a congested high speed area where there is danger of a second accident. If you must, remove the victim feet-first, using three people if possible - one on each side, the other supporting the victim's head and neck.

Follow these rules in examining the patient;

1. Be sure that the victim is breathing and has a pulse (see

pages 18 and 24).

2. Check for hemorrhage (see page 14)
3. Examine for injuries, particularly fractures.
4. Apply appropriate first-aid measures (see index)
5. In case of fractures, wait for medical help. Or, if the person must be moved to get help, follow the suggested procedures for dealing with broken bones (see page 71) and for moving an injured person (see page 37).

BLEEDING - SEVERE

Definition/Diagnosis: The objective with a bleeding wound is to stop the bleeding, treat for shock and transport the victim (or call 911) for definitive care. In remote areas, it may be appropriate for you to provide definitive care yourself.

The first objective is to SAVE THE VICTIM'S LIFE. You do this by stopping the bleeding and treating for shock. Even if the victim is not bleeding badly, you should still treat for shock. Shock has many medical definitions, but what it boils down to is an inadequate amount of oxygen (via the blood) getting to the brain. Lay the patient down, elevate the feet above the head, and provide protection from the environment - from both the ground and the atmosphere. Grab anything you can find for this. (jackets, blankets, etc.). See also Shock on page 39.

To stop bleeding, the keys to remember in this order are:

- Direct Pressure
- Elevation
- Pressure Points
- Tourniquet

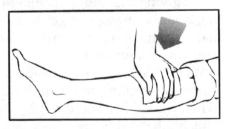

Direct pressure is the best method to stop bleeding. In fact direct pressure alone can stop the bleeding from an amputated limb. When the accident first occurs, you may need to use your bare hand to stem the flow of blood. Ideally, you will have something to protect you from direct contact with the blood and to protect the wound from your dirty hands (admit it your hands are probably dirty). Vinyl gloves are best if you've got them on hand (they store better for long term than latex). If the blood is spurting in rhythm with the beat of the heart, an artery has be severed. This is much more dangerous and the person can bleed out within just a couple of minutes. If arterial bleeding is not stopped quickly, you may need to resort to the use of a tourniquet. If you need to use direct pressure, elevating the limb and pressure points to successfully keep the person from bleeding, keep doing just that. A tourniquet is designed to save the persons life often at the cost of the limb.

Treatment

1. Have the person lie down to prevent fainting. Give the person cayenne tincture in the mouth (1 to 10 dropperfuls). Grab a piece of cloth or whatever you can get a hold of to act as a barrier to stop the bleeding (sterile gauze of course is ideal). Place the gauze or cloth over the wound and with the palm of your hand press it firmly. If severe bleeding from the head or extremities is not controlled within a couple minutes add more material or gauze pads over the existing pads and apply more pressure while holding "pressure points" on major arteries (blood vessels carry blood from the heart to the body).

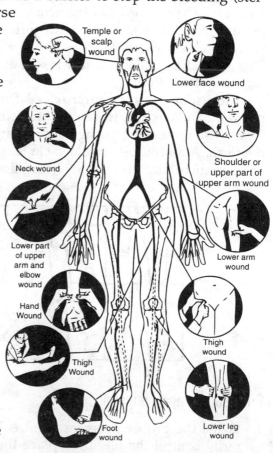

Temple or scalp wound

Lower face wound

Neck wound

Shoulder or upper part of upper arm wound

Lower part of upper arm and elbow wound

Hand Wound

Lower arm wound

Thigh Wound

Thigh wound

Foot wound

Lower leg wound

Applying direct pressure is the surest defense to stopping bleeding. Always use gauze or other clean cloth over the wound.

Apply pressure with thumb and fingers to the major artery supplying blood to the wounded area. If the wound is on the head, neck, arm or leg, and there's no suspected fracture, elevate it - to a level above the heart - to help stop the bleeding while you are applying direct pressure. If you have not given the person a healthy dose of cayenne tincture (1 to 10 dropperfuls) do so immediately. Cayenne stops bleeding.

Also, to help control bleeding along with holding pressure points, elevate the limb that is involved, letting gravity assist in the process. (Caution: If there is a fracture to the limb, use your common sense, taking care with this procedure.) If severe bleeding continues after using the above procedures, with blood spurting from the wound with each heart beat, the use of a tourniquet may be required to save a life (especially in cases where the person has already lost the limb). This should be used as a last resort as it may result in the sacrifice of the limb.

A tourniquet can be improvised from a strap, belt, suspender, handkerchief, towel, necktie, cloth or other material. Never use wire, cord, string or anything that could cut into the flesh. A tourniquet should be at least three to four inches wide to distribute pressure over the tissue.

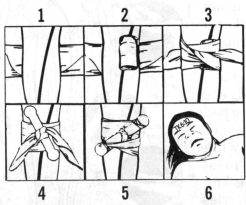

Procedure to apply a tourniquet:

1. While the proper pressure point is being held to temporarily control the bleeding, place the tourniquet between

the heart and the wound with enough uninjured flesh between the wound and the tourniquet. Remember if you are able to control the bleeding using direct pressure points and cayenne, you should not have to apply a tourniquet.

2. Apply a pad (rolled gauze or cloth) over the artery to be compressed (figure #2—opposite page)

3. Wrap the material tightly around the limb (over the pad) twice then tie a half knot (right over left). (figure #3)

4. Place a short stick or similar object at the half knot then complete the knot (left over right). (figure #4)

5. Twist the stick to tighten the tourniquet only until the bleeding stops. If you can stop the bleeding at the wound, while still allowing some circulation to the rest of the arm that is all the better.

6. Secure the stick in place by tying the stick secure with the ends of the cloth. (figure #5)

7. Do not cover the tourniquet. Leave it exposed and visable to others.

8. It is important that you note the time that the tourniquet was applied. Classically you will write this on the persons forehead with a permanent marker (they will not care). This is vital information that should be readily available to emergency personel. (figure #6)

If emergency help is on the way or soon available, do not remove the tourniquet. Removal can cause break through bleeding. The surge of blood will blow right through the clot that has developed, creating a bigger problem. If help is not on its way you may need to loosen the tourniquet every 5 minutes or so while applying direct pressure on the wound to see if adequate bleeding control can be obtained by direct pressure alone. Repeat this as often as necessary. If the bleeding has stopped, the tourniquet can be removed, by slowly releasing pressure then removing. If bleeding has not stopped retighten the tournequet as directed above to stop the bleeding. - it is important that the injured person receive medical attention immediatly.

Herbal Considerations: Internally, use **Cayenne** tincture 10 - 20 drops every few minutes until blood flow stops. You can use 10 dropperfuls of cayenne internally. Cayenne is powerful and should help greatly to control the bleeding. Cayenne is also effective in the treatment of shock. Topically, use **Cayenne** powder directly on the wound - Just pack it in. Shepherd's Purse, Yarrow, Kelp, Plantain, Goldenseal or Horsetail poultice can also be applied directly to the wound or used internally as a tea to help stop the bleeding. Use Herbal Anti-Septic Tincture once the bleeding has stopped and before you begin to bandage. (See Cleaning a Wound, page 199.)

When the bleeding stops, bandage the dressings firmly in place, but not so tight that you can't feel the pulse below or beyond the wound. Call the paramedics or your doctors and defer to them for final treatment and cleaning of the wound.

Watch carefully for signs of shock (see page 39).

How to Make a Bandage: Bandages can be made from most any cloth or material, as illustrated with the T-shirt.

To prevent infection, avoid, if possible, touching any wound with an unsterilized covering or your unscrubbed hands. In an emergency, you may have no choice. The average adult has five to six quarts of blood; loss of more than two pints can be serious. It is important to act fast and use whatever supplies and resources are available. Once the situation has calmed down, it may be important to assist the patient in drinking fluids (water with a pinch of sea salt) to replace any blood that may have been lost. Do not force fluids on anyone that is not fully conscious.

BREATHING STOPPED -
Artificial Respiration/also called Rescue Breathing

The cessation of breathing is a medical emergency requiring immediate treatment. The following steps should be taken immediately:

1. Have someone call 911.

2. Open the airway. Make sure the air passageway is cleared of any obstructions, either solid or liquid. Remove any foreign objects from the mouth or nose. This includes false teeth, dentures, bridges, etc.

3. Place the palm of one hand on the forehead and tip the person's head back extending the neck to maximize the airway. Place the fingers of the other hand under the chin and lift to bring it forward. (See illustration at right) Do not overextend the neck or tip the head back if the neck is injured. This position prevents obstruction of the airway by the tongue. (When the lower jaw falls downward in an unconscious person, the tongue also falls back, obstructing the throat.) Opening the airway

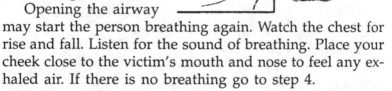

may start the person breathing again. Watch the chest for rise and fall. Listen for the sound of breathing. Place your cheek close to the victim's mouth and nose to feel any exhaled air. If there is no breathing go to step 4.

4. Pinch the nostrils closed with your thumb and finger that is resting on the victim's forehead. To do this, maneuver your hand so that it continues to exert the necessary pressure on the head to maintain the proper tilt. Place your mouth over the victim's mouth and give two full breaths, taking a deep gulp of air in between the two. Each ventilation should cause the victim's chest to rise and fall. If this fails to happen, try adjusting the victim's head, and repeat the two full breaths. If this, too, fails to expand the chest and lungs, suspect an obstruction in the airway. See instructions for choking. (page 27).

    When you are able to get air into the victim's lung quickly proceed to step 5.

5. Feel the carotid pulse. It is not difficult to locate the ca-

rotid pulse. [It can be felt on either side of the neck. Locate the Adam's apple (the larynx), then slide the tips of your index and middle fingers gently into the groove between the Adam's apple and the muscles of the neck. Practice locating your own carotid pulse. Don't compress the pulse area - touch it softly.] Feel for the pulse for 5 to 10 seconds. (See illustration on previous page). If there is no pulse, begin performing CPR (next section). If there is a pulse but still no breathing, begin step 6 - steady mouth-to-mouth breathing.

6. With the victim's head tilted as in step 1, and his nose pinched shut, place your mouth over the victim's and blow hard. Remove your mouth to allow the victim to exhale and you to take another breath. Watch for the rise and fall of the chest and listen for the sound of exhaled air. Then blow again. Repeat this procedure, giving one vigorous breath every five seconds until the victim starts to breathe on his own or until help arrives.

Have someone call 911 immediately. Place a blanket or coat over the person for warmth if necessary. If the person revives, don't let him get up. Keep him lying down and resting until help arrives.

For infants and small children, the procedure is modified. By definition an infant is age 0 to 1 and a child is from age 1 to 8 years. To open the airway, avoid over-extension of the child's head as this will cause the airway to close. Lift the chin only slightly, using one or two fingers. Leave the other hand on the forehead to keep the head in the proper position. Do not pinch the nose closed but cover the mouth and nose with your mouth. Gently give two slow breaths - use only light puffs of air to inflate a child's lungs. Feel the pulse (inside the upper arm between elbow and shoulder for infants - slide off the biceps muscle then roll up onto the arm bone- the humorous). If there is a pulse, give one gentle puff of air once every three seconds for an infant, every four seconds for a child.

If you suspect a victim's neck is broken, avoid all movement of the neck. To open the airway, place a hand on each side of the victim's head to maintain it in a neutral position. Then use the index fingers to move the lower jaw forward, without moving the head or neck. (It may be easier to use mouth-to-nose respiration. Place your cheek over the victim's mouth and breath into his nose.)

NOTE: If there is no response, check airway again for foreign objects. If a pulse cannot be found, administer CPR (Cardio-Pulmonary Resuscitation).

Herbal Considerations: Lobelia tincture is used to help a person breathe easier and open up the airway. If the person is conscious use 2 to 10 dropperfuls in the mouth. If the person is unconscious use 1 to 2 dropperfuls in the mouth. A dropperful is measured by one squeeze of the bulb and should be about 30 drops. Cayenne tincture can be used to revive a heart attack.

BURNS

Grease - Remove all grease from burn with soap and water. Submerge burned area in cold water, or burns that cannot be submerged in water cover with a wet, cold towel, changing them frequently. Once the area is clean and has been submerged or soaked in cold water for 45 minutes to one hour, apply CTR Ointment or Dr. Christopher's Burn Ointment (Equal parts wheat germ oil, honey, and comfrey leaf). Reapply ointment 3 times per day keeping covered with sterile gauze. When applying fresh ointment do not remove existing ointment. It will be absorbed and the nutrients utilized by the body to heal the damaged tissue in that area. Use Immune Boost internally 1 to 2 dropperfuls, three times daily to ward against infection.

Chemical - Flush the burned area many times with tepid water to dilute and remove the chemical for as long a 15-20 minutes. Baking soda mixed with water or Olive oil can be used to neutralize the burn. Treat herbally the same as you would other burns.

If an eye is burned by a chemical, especially an acid or an alkaline substance like lye, flush it at once gently but thoroughly with tepid running water for 15 minutes. Cover both eyes with gauze or a clean cloth. (otherwise, when the uninjured eye moves, the injured eye will also move, so cover both eyes). Have the eye checked at once by a doctor.

Burns and Scalds - Minor

Submerge the burned area **immediately** in cold water or apply cold, wet towels. On burns that cannot be immersed, apply cloths soaked in ice water, and change them constantly. Avoid greases and baking soda, especially on burns severe enough to require medical treatment. Doctors must always scrape off such applications, which delays treatment and can be extremely painful. If the skin is blistered, cover with sterile dressings. Do not break or drain blisters.

Treatment: Aloe vera is the best burn treatment. Fillet a frond of aloe vera and apply the slab of clear aloe vera. Secure with gauze or a bandage and replace with the next slab of aloe vera. Apply Olive Oil or Vitamin E Oil to help with healing and to prevent pulling when bandages are changed. Apply CTR (Complete Tissue Repair) Ointment (page 224-225) or Dr. Christopher's Burn Ointment (equal part comfrey, wheat germ oil, and honey) until completely healed, add new ointment every four hours. Do not try to remove old ointment, just keep adding ointment to the wound. Cover the burn with a sterile dressing or clean sheet. This reduces exposure to the open air reducing pain and the risk of contamination.

Use Immune Boost internally, 2 dropperfuls 6 times daily.

For sunburns, apple cider vinegar, Aloe vera, cucumber or CTR ointment may be used successfully for pain relief and to speed recovery without peeling.

Burns and Scalds - Major

1. If the victim's clothing is on fire, or still smoldering, stop the burning by rolling him on the ground. Douse him with

water or smother the flames with a coat, blanket or rug.

2. Keep the victim lying down, to lessen shock. Treat person for shock as may be necessary.

3. Cut around all clothing that has adhered to the skin (do not try to pull it loose). Cool with water.

4. Call 911 immediately or move the victim to the nearest hospital.

5. Do not apply any oils, ointments, etc. prior to transporting the patient to the hospital. The medical community will not understand your attempts as an herbalist and will be only alarmed and irritated at what you have done, as they vigorously scrub the raw skin to remove it. Use only water. Lots and lots of water.

6. If hospital and professional help can not be part of the treatment plan (severe burns that cover large portions of the body, you should get help!) then use the following herbal therapies. Healing the tissue with herbs really is the treatment of choice, however, with third degree burns over large areas, lifesaving efforts may need to be employed.

7. Use cayenne pepper orally to prevent shock (1-2 dropperfuls) and lobelia tincture after 15 minutes to help the person relax and to help ease the pain.

8. Aloe vera is the best burn treatment. Fillet (peel) a frond(the leaf) of aloe vera and apply the slab of clear aloe vera. Secure with gauze or a bandage and replace with the next slab of aloe vera.

9. Apply CTR Ointment and Dr. Christopher's Burn Ointment (equal part comfrey, wheat germ oil, and honey) until completely healed, add new ointment every four hours. Do not try to remove old ointment, just keep adding ointment to the wound. Cover the burn with a sterile dressing or clean sheet. This reduces exposure to the open air reducing pain and the risk of contamination.

10. Use Immune Boost internally, 2 dropperfuls 6 times daily.

11. Applying Olive Oil (always use extra virgin) or Vitamin E Oil will help with healing and to prevent pulling when bandages are changed.

CPR (CARDIO-PULMONARY RESUSCITATION)
Breathing Stopped, No Pulse

Definition/Diagnosis: CPR should only be administered when breathing has stopped and there is no pulse. Check the carotid artery (side of the neck) carefully as the pulse may be weak. If there is a heartbeat but no sign of breathing, perform artificial respiration.

Caution on Cardiopulmonary resuscitation:

This lifesaving technique requires training, skill and practice. The untrained may cause serious damage to the patient. To be prepared for an emergency, at least one member of every family should seek instruction from the local Red Cross, Heart Association, or other local agencies. Ask your local Fire Department or Hospital where to go.

Note: Without CPR, anyone whose heart has stopped will die, so in an emergency it may be necessary to perform CPR even if you are untrained.

Treatment: Remember the ABC's (see page 1). Make certain that the airway is clear; give two full breaths, and feel the carotid pulse (see previous section, page 18-19).

If there is no pulse, the heart has stopped. While someone calls for an ambulance, CPR must be started at once. CPR is the combination of artificial respiration and artificial circulation - externally compression the chest.

Procedure for CPR

1. Have someone call 911.

2. With the victim stretched flat on their back on the ground or the floor, kneel beside him and position their head to keep the chin up and the airway open (see illustration). Give the patient two full breaths. This will confirm that the airway is established and there is no obstruction.

3. Give cayenne tincture orally (1 to 2 dropperfuls). If the person is unconscious, cayenne will increase the circulation and can revive someone from a heart attack. With any emergency or critical situation do not over look support for the rescuer. A dropperful of cayenne can benefit the rescuer as well.

4. Feel the chest to locate the lower tip of the victim's breastbone (see illustration on previous page). Place two fingers of your left hand on the tip. Then move the heel of your right hand (never the palm) above (headward) the fingers on the lower breastbone. The heel of your right hand should be about 1 - 1 1/2 inches above the tip and over the lower third of the breastbone. Then place the left hand on top of the right. For adults and children over 80 pounds only, place heel of hand on the persons lower breast bone. Clasp fingers and bend those of lower hand back.(If you are left-handed, reverse the hand instructions).

5. Position your body so that your shoulders are directly above your hands, with arms straight and elbow locked (see illustration page 26).

6. With a smooth, firm thrust, push down. Use sufficient force to press the lower one-third of the breastbone down at least 1 to 1 1/2 inches, letting your back and body do the work. (You are pressing the breastbone against the heart forcing it to contract and pump the blood.) Then lift your weight, relaxing pressure completely.

7. Do not remove your hands from the victim's chest when you relax between compression's. Never press the tip of the breastbone. Do not allow your fingers to press on the chest. If you interlock your fingers this is easier.

8. Repeat this rhythmic compression - press...release...press... release - 15 times at a rate of 80 - 100 times a minute (this is more than one compression every second). Then give two full breaths into the mouth of the victim, breathing like you would during artificial respiration. Continue this 15 to 2 rhythm four times. Check the pulse for five seconds. If no pulse, resume CPR, reassessing the patient every five minutes. Repeat the 15 to 2 cycle until a pulse is felt or person revives. At this rate you should be breathing for the patient about 8-10 times during each minute. If a pulse

returns, but there is no breathing, continue with artificial respiration at a rate of 12 breaths per minute. That is one breath every 5 seconds. Count out loud and keep a steady rhythm.

9. To help maintain proper timing, count out loud in this style: "one-and, two-and, three-and. . ." until you have done the required 15 compression's.

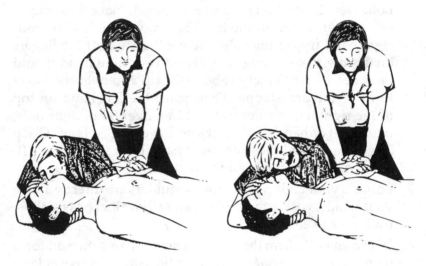

CPR for Infants and Small Children

Clear the airway and check for a pulse. Refer to special instructions for artificial respiration for children. Cayenne pepper (a few drops) can be used to stimulate the circulation and can save a life. For chest compression, use only the tip of the index and middle fingers on one hand. Use your judgment on how much of your hand/fingers to use for compression based on the size of the child. For an 60-80 pound child you may use the heel of one hand. For an infant, only finger tips. For infants under one year old, the compression rate is a least 100 times per minute. Use the heel of one hand or as many fingers as are necessary to press down the breastbone. Press down on the area right between the infants nipples. Depress the breastbone 1/2 to 1 inch. Deliver one small breath after each five compressions.

CHOKING
Obstructed Airway

Definition/Diagnosis: The Heimlich maneuver (also called the Abdominal Thrust) is the most effective first-aid measure for choking. Choking means that something - food or a foreign body - is plugging the victims windpipe so that they cannot breathe. If the airway is completely blocked, the victim, unless relieved of the obstruction, may die in less than five minutes. You must act fast.

A leading cause of death in the home is obstruction of the throat or air passage by a foreign object (or choking). Most of these deaths occur among children under the age of 4 who either place an object in their mouth or are given food too large or hard for them to eat.

Treatment: First make certain that the person is choking and not having a heart attack. If a person is eating and suddenly looks startled, puts his hand to his throat, can't speak, talk or breathe, face turns blue, quickly ask him if he is choking. If he is unable to speak and nods his head "Yes", apply the Heimlich maneuver. Lobelia tincture can be used to relax and help open the airway. Use 2 to 10 dropperfuls if the person is conscious and 1 to 2 dropperfuls if the person is unconscious.

To apply **the Heimlich maneuver:** If the victim is sitting or standing, stand up behind him and extend both arms around his waist (see illustration below).

Make a fist with one hand placing the thumb-side against the victim's abdomen, above the navel and below the rib cage.

Grasp your fist with the other hand and thrust your fist upward and back into person's abdomen. Repeat four times or until the object is dislodged. If this doesn't work, place the person on their side and, using the heel of your hand, hit sharply on their spin between the shoulder blades. Repeat the Heimlich maneuver again.

(The Heimlich maneuver works on the principle that there is always some residual air trapped in the lungs of the victim. When compressed by pressure below the diaphragm and forced upward, the air ejects the obstruction caught in the windpipe.)

Caution: Don't squeeze the person with your arms. This could damage the ribs. To avoid squeezing, keep your arms bent at the elbows.

If the person is lying face down, position them face up on their back and kneel astride their thighs. With one of your hands on top of the other, place the heel of your bottom hand on the abdomen between the navel and rib cage. Press with a quick upward thrust. (see illustration page 27).

If you are alone and choking - use your fist to perform the maneuver on yourself, placing the thumb-side of the fist of one hand against the abdomen just above the navel and grasping the fist with the other hand. Or try anything that will apply upward force just below your diaphragm. Lean forward and press into the edge of a table, the kitchen sink, or the back of a chair or doorknob, for example.

If an infant is choking, have someone call 911 while you use the following technique recommended by the American Academy of Pediatrics, American Red Cross and the American Heart Association.

Caution: Do not apply any measures if the child can breathe, speak or make sounds, and is coughing. These signs mean they are getting air in their windpipe that can expel the object partially blocking the airway. Any maneuvers by you can interfere with this natural process and may convert the partial blockage to a total obstruction. Watch closely, but don't interfere.

1. If the choking infant is unable to breathe or make a sound, place the baby face down over your forearm (with the infant's head lower than the rest of the body). Using the heel of your hand, give forceful but measured blows on the baby's back between the shoulder blades.

2. If the back blows fail to eject the object from the wind-

pipe, apply four rapid chest thrusts. To do this: Turn the baby over on their back. Position them on your thighs with their head lower than their torso.

3. Using only the index and middle fingers of one hand, place your fingers on the center of the baby's chest just below the level of the nipples, and compress the chest four times in rapid succession.

4. If the procedure is not successful, open the airway by grasping the tongue and lower jaw between the thumb and finger, and lift. (This draws the tongue away from the back of the throat and may help relieve the obstruction.) Look for a foreign body in the victim's throat. Attempt to remove a foreign body only if it's plainly visible.

    If no spontaneous breathing occurs, deliver two breaths through the mouth or mouth-nose (as in artificial respiration, page 18). If the chest fails to rise, repeat the sequence of back blows and chest thrusts while having someone call for help and emergency transport to a medical facility, or for a rescue unit to come to your home. CPR may be necessary (see page 24).

5. To rescue a small child who is choking, place the victim face up on the floor and proceed as recommended for an adult victim lying down, except kneel at the feet of the child. Use both hands to administer the Heimlich maneuver (abdominal thrust), placing the heel of the underneath hand on the child's abdomen between the navel and the rib cage. Apply the thrust gently.

DIABETIC COMA and INSULIN REACTION
(or Insulin Shock)

Definition/Diagnosis: If someone becomes confused, incoherent or unconscious for no apparent reason, he may be having an insulin reaction or developing a diabetic coma.

Insulin reaction is the result of a too-rapid drop in the diabetic's blood-sugar level. The diabetic sweats profusely and is nervous; his pulse is rapid, his breathing is shallow. He may be hazy and faltering, or appear drunk. If he is conscious and can swallow, give him some form of sugar - candy, sugar cubes, fruit juice or a sweet soft drink. **No artificially sweetened products.** If recovery is not prompt, or if the diabetic cannot swallow or is unconscious, call for emergency medical assistance.

The symptoms of diabetic coma come on gradually. It is frequently preceded by excessive urination. The diabetics' skin becomes flushed and dry, the tongue dry, behavior drowsy, breathing labored; breath develops a fruity odor. Diabetic coma requires prompt medical attention and emergency hospitalization.

When in doubt give the patient something sweet as it will quickly turn an insulin reaction around and will do little to worsen a diabetic headed towards coma.

Garlic is an ideal herb to balance and correct blood sugar levels. Any person with diabetes can take 6 or more cloves of garlic daily. Other herbs helpful for diabetes are cedar berries, devils club and Gymnema

HYPOGLYCEMIA

Definition/Diagnosis: This condition is caused by the blood sugar dropping too low. Most often it is the result of too much insulin being released by the pancreas. A person suffering from hypoglycemia may suffer from any or all of the following symptoms: fatigue, dizziness, lightheadedness, shakiness, headache, irritability, fainting spells, depression, anxiety, craving for sweets, confusion, night sweats, weakness in legs, swollen feet, a feeling of tightness in the chest, constant hunger, pain in various parts of the body especially the eyes, nervousness, quick temper and aggressiveness. The liver is involved in blood sugar regulation.

Treatment: An acute episode can be simply resolved by eating or drinking something that will increase the blood sugar. If hypoglycemia is found in a diabetic patient refer to "Diabetic Coma and Insulin Reaction" (page 29). If this is a chronic problem for a non-diabetic consult with your healthcare practitioner. A liver flush and cleansing the liver is important for overcoming chronic hypoglycemia. (see page 257-259)

DROWNING

If the victim is not breathing, clear the airway and start artificial respiration at once (see page 18-21). Administer CPR if the heart has stopped (see page 24). Take special care if a broken neck is suspected (see page 76). Remember cayenne pepper is used to revive and lobelia is used to aid in breathing. These are two herbs that you should always have on hand.

EPILEPTIC SEIZURE, CONVULSION

Definition/Diagnosis: Seizures can be the result of many different conditions from epilepsy, drug reactions, poisoning, hypoglycemia to prolonged high fever.

Treatment: Call 911. If possible, turn the person having a seizure on to one side. Don't try to restrain convulsive movement. Move furniture or nearby objects that might cause injury while the person is making involuntary movements. Don't put anything in the person's mouth. The seizure usually ends within a few minutes. When it ends, the person may experience some confusion. Reassure him and assist him in obtaining further medical help. When the seizure is over treat the person appropriately if poisoned, hypoglycemic etc. Herbally use lobelia tincture under the tongue, once the seizure has stopped. Two to ten dropperfuls of lobelia should be administered orally as soon as you are able. Calcium Tea and Nerve Calm are effective to calm the muscles down. Herbs that have been effective in reducing the frequency and intensity of seizures are Ashwaganda, Black Cohosh, Blue Cohosh, Lobelia and Motherwort.

FAINTING

Treatment: Place the person on their back. Make certain that their airway is clear and that they are breathing. Loosen tight clothing and elevate their legs; apply cold cloths to their face.

If the fainting lasts more than a minute or two, keep the person covered if necessary to maintain normal body temperature, and call an ambulance or take them to the hospital.

Fainting may be caused by fatigue, hunger, sudden emotional upset, a poorly ventilated room, etc. The person's breathing is usually weak, pulse feeble, face pale and forehead covered with beads of perspiration. If the person merely feels faint, have them lie down or at least sit with their head lowered to their knees.

Cayenne pepper will get the blood to the brain quicker

than anything. If a person begins to look or feel faint, give them cayenne and that will generally pull them out of it.

HEAD INJURY
Fracture, Concussion

Definition/Diagnosis: There is the possibility of head injury in any auto accident, fall or other incident of violence. The brain is only about one millimeter from the inside of your skull. That's about the thickness of a dime. The fluid (cerebrospinal fluid) within the brain does have some shock absorption ability, but any significant trauma can cause the brain to smash against the skull (and most of us have pretty hard heads). If the brain begins to swell from this trauma, it can create a lot of pressure because the swelling is contained in a tightly closed space. Symptoms may include: becoming dazed or unconscious; rapid but weak pulse; bleeding from mouth, nose or ears; pupils of eyes unequal size; paralysis of one or more extremities; headaches or dizziness; double vision; vomiting; pale skin. Caution: the victim may also appear quite normal and have a momentary loss of consciousness or a lack of memory of the event causing the injury - only to lapse into unconsciousness later, or develop other symptoms.

Head injuries are divided into four categories:

1) **NO LOSS OF CONSCIOUSNESS:** There is only a rare chance of serious problems even though there may have been heavy bleeding and a huge bump or goose-egg. Without loss of consciousness you are generally assured the brain has not been damaged.

2) **MILD OR SHORT-TERM UNCONSCIOUSNESS:** This results when the brain briefly contacted the inside of the skull and some temporary loss of function occurred. Usually short-term unconsciousness is nothing to worry about. Often the victim will be unaware that they lost consciousness. Ask a witness, if possible. Watch for the signs of intracranial pressure (ICP). a) a headache that increases in intensity, b) complaints of blurred vision, c) a decreasing level of consciousness from disoriented to irritable to combative to coma, d) a heart rate that slows down and then starts to bound, e) irregular breathing, often with deep

sighing breaths, f) the face becomes flush and warm, g) increase in blood pressure, h) pupils are unequal in size and do not constrict normally with light.

3) **LONG TERM UNCONSCIOUSNESS:** This is a serious sign that intracranial pressure is on the rise. The problem can be a bruise to the brain, or a tear in the blood vessels of the of the meninges (membranes or lining of the brain), or a tear / laceration to the brain itself. Often there can be a pooling of blood within the brain called a subdural hematoma. This blood clot can increase in size over hour or weeks increasing the pressure in the brain resulting in permanent damage or death.

4) **OBVIOUS HEAD INJURIES:** This would include obvious fractures where you may see a depression in the skull or a visible fracture line where a portion of the scalp may be torn away, black and blue around swollen eyes (Raccoon eyes), black and blue behind and below the ears (Battle's sign), and blood or clear cerebrospinal fluid (or both mixed) leaking from the nose or ears. Seizures with these kind of injuries are common.

Treatment: If the victim is unconscious, check breathing and pulse. Perform artificial respiration (see page 18) or CPR (see page 24) if necessary. If these steps are not needed and no neck or back injury is suspected, turn the victim on his side so that blood or mucus can drain from the corner of the mouth. Get medical assistance at once. Call 911. Always treat the most serious or life threatening condition first. With obvious head injuries you should assume that there is also an injury to the cervical spine.

Even though the person may look OK, there is always danger of brain hemorrhage and serious trouble later. Lying quietly lessens the chance of hemorrhage. If the scalp is bleeding, place a dressing over the wound and bandage it into place. Keep the person lying down until you get medical help. If you must leave them alone for any reason, roll them carefully on their side to ensure that the airway remains open. The head-injured are prone to vomiting, often multiple times. Aspirated vomitus (vomit sucked into the lungs) usually causes death. Keep them lying down, on a slope if possible, with their head slightly uphill. Gravity can help to reduce the swelling in the brain. The patient has the greatest chance for survival with hospital treatment, with the use of oxygen therapy, surgery and drugs. While the person is in your care arouse them regularly. If you cannot arouse them, then it is time for outside help. If getting to help is no an immediate option, you may let the person sleep as the brain while sleeping will have the best chance of controlling it's own swelling. Prognosis is very good if the person shows signs of improvement within 48 hours.

Cayenne pepper can be used to assist with any external or internal bleeding, as well as to rouse a person back into consciousness if they begin to drift away. Herbally, you can put a dropperful of cayenne tincture under the tongue of the person, even if unconscious to help stop bleeding and internal hemorrhaging. Comfrey is known to both heal and reduce inflammation. A comfrey fomentation wrapped around the head can be used. CTR syrup is beneficial for healing wounds internally (see page 224). Once the person is out of immediate crisis or is at least stabilized direction of energy technique can be used (see page 263).

HEART ATTACK
Myocardial Infarction

Definition/Diagnosis: The symptoms of chest heaviness or pain with exertion; pain or ache radiating into the neck or into the arms; sweating, clammy, pale appearance; and/or shortness of breath are fairly classic for a person having an inadequate oxygen supply to the heart. The pain is called "angina" and results from the heart muscle starving for oxygen, just as a cramp or "Charlie horse" is the pain of a muscle screaming for oxygen. If the blockage is severe, the heart muscle will die. This is called a "myocardial infarction" and it means heart attack and damaged muscle. The cause of death is frequently a profound irregular heart beat caused by electrical irritation in the damaged muscle. Another cause of death is loss of adequate power to pump blood from weakened heart muscles. A delayed cause of death can be from the sudden rupture of the weakened heart wall.

Treatment: Do not ignore the symptoms of a heart attack. Call 911 immediately. Have the person lie down and rest. If the person is having trouble breathing, do not force him to lie down. Help him take the position that is most comfortable for him. Loosen tight clothing. Don't attempt to lift or carry him. Herbally, give the person 1 to 10 dropperfuls of Cayenne tincture orally. Often the cayenne is enough to pull someone out of an acute heart attack before any permanent damage to the heart is done. Even if the person is unconscious 1 to 2 dropperfuls of cayenne can be put into the mouth. Rest causes the oxygen requirement of the heart to be at a minimum. Don't give him anything to drink. Remain calm, and try to reassure him. Observe the respiration and pulse rates. Rehearse in your mind the steps in CPR (see page 24) in case the person loses his pulse and stops breathing. Be prepared to perform CPR if necessary. Deep Heat ointment or oil can be massaged on the persons arm.

For Long Term care for people with a history or predisposition of heart concerns whether it be previous heart attack, angina, palpitations or arrhythmia's use Hawthorn Berry Syrup and Heart Formula, and Motherwort. These herbs will assist in more efficient utilization of oxygen with the heart and red blood cells. A formula made of 1 part cayenne and 3 parts hawthorn(berry, leaf and/or flowers) is a good heart tonic that can begin during a heart attack and as part of the recovery. Hawthorn is a heart protector.

Often high cholesterol is associated with heart and circulatory disease. To lower cholesterol, one must focus on cleansing and flushing the liver. Once the liver is "unclogged", the cholesterol will come down. Of course diet and exercise is important, but without proper liver function, the cholesterol will not come down. Emphasizing soy proteins such as tofu, Miso, soy cheese and Tamari are shown to help reduce cholesterol.

ANEMIA

Anemia is the reduction of the number of red blood cells in the blood. Anemia reduces the oxygen carrying capacity of the blood resulting in fatigue, lethargy and dizziness. The anemic person will often appear very pale and when shining a light behind the ears (looking at the color of the ear with the light behind), it will not be as red as someone who in not anemic. Build the blood with chlorophyll. Chlorophyll is similar in structure to hemoglobin, which carries the oxygen in the red blood cells. Take SuperNutrition 2 - 3 times daily. Yellow dock tincture can be taken as a very rich source of natural iron. Blackstrap molasses is a good source of iron and essential B vitamins. If anemia persists see your healthcare practitioner, as there are many causes of anemia.

BLOOD PRESSURE
(High or Low)

Definition/Diagnosis: This cannot be determined without the use of a blood pressure cuff and stethoscope. If you are in a situation where you are taking the blood pressure but there is too much background noise, rather than listening for the returning pulse as you loosen the pressure, feel for the first pulse at the wrist. This will be you systolic pressure.

Treatment: The liver needs to be flushed and "unclogged", as well as the colon. High blood pressure associated with high cholesterol requires cleansing the liver, the colon and changing the diet. Cayenne tincture or powder (10-15 drops, or 1/2 to 1 tsp.) 2 times daily. Shepherd's Purse Tincture 10-20 drops 2 times daily. Three to six cloves of fresh garlic is advisable. Lobelia Tincture to lower blood pressure 3-5 drops 2 times daily. Follow a Vegetarian (High complex Carbohydrates, Low Fat and Protein) diet. Emphasize fresh fruits and vegetables.

HEART RATE
Rapid (Tachycardia)

Definition/Diagnosis: A rapid heart rate after trauma or other stress may signify impending shock. The underlying cause should be treated. This may require fluid replacement or herbs for pain. Body temperature elevations cause an increase in heart rate of 10 beats per minute for each degree above normal. At elevations above 8,000 feet (2,500 meter), a pulse rate of 120 or greater after 20 minutes of rest is an early sign of pulmonary edema. A sudden onset of rapid heart rate with sharp chest pain can indicate a pulmonary embolism or pneumothorax.

A very rapid heart rate/ pulse rate of 140 to 220 beats per minute may be encountered suddenly and without warning in very healthy persons. This PAT (paroxysmal arterial Tachy-cardia) has as its first symptom, frequently, a feeling of profound weakness.

Treatment: The victim generally stops what they are doing and feels better sitting sown. These attacks are self-limited, by they can be aborted by one of the several maneuvers which stimulate the vagus nerve which in turn slows down the pulse rate. These maneuvers include; holding one's breath and bearing down very hard, closing one's eyes and pressing firmly on the eyeballs; inducing vomiting with a finger down the throat; or feeling for the carotid pulse in the neck and gently pressing on the enlarged portion of this vessel, one side at a time. Frequently, however, the victim must just wait for the attack to pass. This arrhythmia will sometimes come on after increase in activity. Herbally, lobelia (1 to 5 dropperfuls) can be taken internally. Use Motherwort herb 3-4 times daily for continued palpitations, or a weak and nervous heart.

HEART RATE
Slow (Bradycardia)

Definition/Diagnosis: A slow heart rate is important in two instances: when associated with passing out and when accompanied by high fever. Generally fainting or shock is associated with a rapid pulse rate (see compensatory shock, page 39). When the blood pressure rises to a certain point however, there is a protective mechanism which prevents the blood pressure from rising too high causing the heart rate and blood pressure to slow and lower. The resulting slow pulse and relaxed arteries result in the person passing out.

The pulse rate can also lower as the core body temperature lowers as in hypothermia. There are several diseases that the pulse rate is lower than would be expected for the elevated body temperature caused by the disease. One example of this would by typhoid fever. Cayenne pepper is the greatest circulatory stimulant and is the herb of choice for most circulatory concerns.

MOVING AN INJURED PERSON

If an injury involves the neck or back, damage can be done

by moving the victim. Get a doctor or ambulance quickly, if possible; meanwhile, cover the patient with blankets or coats if necessary to maintain body temperature. Do not attempt to change his position until you determine the nature of his injuries - unless it is absolutely necessary to prevent further injuries. If the victim must be pulled to safety, move his body lengthwise (not sideways) and headfirst, with his head and neck carefully supported. If possible, slip a blanket or long coat under him so he can ride on that. If the person must be lifted, don't lift him by his heels and head only. This bends the body at the waist which can further injuries. Support each part of the body so that you lift it in a straight line as if the person were lying on a board.

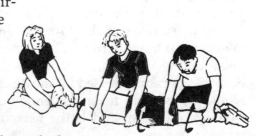

Until you are certain that there is no neck or back injury, don't bundle a seriously injured person into an automobile and speed to the nearest town. If a victim must be transported, move him in a reclining or semi-reclining position. Improvise a stretcher, if possible. The most desirable is a door or wide board. Lacking either of these, make a stretcher out of blankets and poles, or out of buttoned jackets with the sleeves turned inward and the poles running through the sleeves. If the victim is conscious, and not suffering from back, neck or leg injuries, use a chair (carried by two or more persons) to bring him down narrow or winding stairs.

When reporting an accident, inform the doctor or ambulance service of the nature of the accident and injuries. Seek advice regarding the safest procedure.

SHOCK

Definition/Diagnosis: Shock is the deficiency of oxygen reaching the brain and other tissues as a result of decreased circulation. An important aspect of the correction of shock is to identify and treat the underlying cause. Shock can be caused by burns, electrocution, hypothermia, bites, stings, bleeding, fractures, pain, hypothermia, high altitude cerebral edema, illness, rough handling, allergic reactions (anaphy-

SIGNS AND SYMPTOMS OF SHOCK

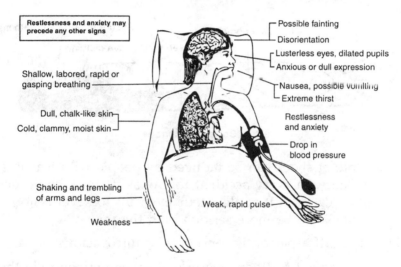

Restlessness and anxiety may precede any other signs

Shallow, labored, rapid or gasping breathing

Dull, chalk-like skin
Cold, clammy, moist skin

Shaking and trembling of arms and legs

Weakness

Possible fainting
Disorientation
Lusterless eyes, dilated pupils
Anxious or dull expression

Nausea, possible vomiting
Extreme thirst

Restlessness and anxiety

Drop in blood pressure

Weak, rapid pulse

laxis), damage or excitement of the central nervous system, dehydration from sweating, vomiting or diarrhea, or loss of adequate heart strength. Each of these underlying causes is discussed separately in this text.

Shock can progress through several stages before death result. The first phase is called the "COMPENSATORY STAGE" during which the body attempts to counter the damage by increasing its activity level. Arteries constrict and the pulse rate increase, thus maintaining the blood pressure. The next phase is called the "PROGRESSIVE STAGE" when suddenly the blood pressure drops and the patient becomes worse, often swiftly. When they have reached the "IRREVERSIBLE STAGE" vital organs have suffered from loss of oxygen so profoundly that death occurs even with aggressive treatment.

Consider the possibility of shock in any victim or an accident or when significant illness develops. Make sure adequate airways are opened. Assess the cardiovascular status. If the pulse rate is over 140 in adults or 180 in children they may be in the compensatory stage of shock.

Check blood pressure, shallow rapid breathing, nausea and vomiting. Often the patient will be frightened. Also watch for partial or complete loss of consciousness.

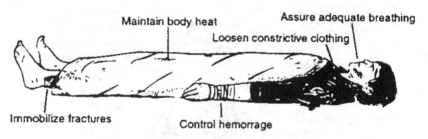

Reassure patient
Position patient
Relieve pain

Maintain body heat

Assure adequate breathing

Loosen constrictive clothing

Immobilize fractures

Control hemorrage

A state of shock can be induced by people with fear in a minor injury. In every accident follow as if shock could occur and treat as if it could occur even up to several hours later. Shock can be more serious than the injury.

Treatment: If a person is conscious or unconscious:

1. Administer 1 to 10 dropperfuls of cayenne tincture in the mouth. Shepherds purse tincture can be substituted but is a distant second to cayenne.

2. Lie the person flat on their back, with legs elevated to insure a better venous return of blood to the heart and head. In cases of head or chest injury, when the patient has difficulty breathing, the head and shoulders should be raised so that the head is 10 inches higher than the feet.

3. Make sure the person is warm - replace any wet clothing. Loosen any tight or restrictive clothing. A person in mild shock can still produce body heat. A person in severe shock

loses the ability to produce body heat. When this happens, no amount of clothing will help to restore body heat. Hypothermia and irreversible shock then takes place, and the person can die. In severe shock, external heat needs to be applied. The best heat source is from another person, one or more, to come in contact skin to skin in sleeping bags (like a cocoon) with the person in shock.

4. Internally, keep administering cayenne tincture and nettle tincture to improve circulation and produce internal heat. All future heat loss to the person in extreme shock should be avoided.

STROKE

Definition/Diagnosis: A stroke is a life threatening injury in which an artery in the brain becomes clogged by a blood clot or ruptures. The resulting disruption of blood flow cuts off the oxygen supply to the part of the brain which is downstream from the injury. In a sense, a stroke is similar to a heart attack, except the arterial blockage occurs in the brain rather than the heart. If a blood clot becomes dislodged and blocks an artery in the heart, a heart attack ensues. If the same clot clogs an artery in the brain, it is a stroke. A stroke can effect the senses, speech, behavior, thought patterns and memory. It can also result in paralysis, coma and death. Signs and symptoms of a stroke include:

- Severe headache
- Convulsions (seizures)
- Change in the level of mental ability
- Consciousness or alertness is decreased
- Change in personality
- Pupils unequal in size
- Loss or a dimness of vision
- Drooping mouth or eyelids (usually on one side only)
- A Sudden weakness or paralysis of face, arm or leg.
- Inability to speak
- Understanding speech is difficult for patient
- Paralysis or weakness on one or both sides of the body (usually one side only)

- Pulse is rapid and strong
- Difficulty breathing (respiratory distress)
- Loss of bowel or bladder control
- Nausea and/or vomiting

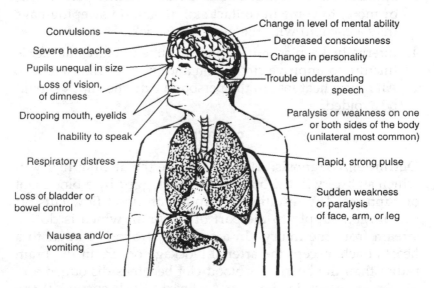

Convulsions

Severe headache

Pupils unequal in size

Loss of vision, of dimness

Drooping mouth, eyelids

Inability to speak

Respiratory distress

Loss of bladder or bowel control

Nausea and/or vomiting

Change in level of mental ability

Decreased consciousness

Change in personality

Trouble understanding speech

Paralysis or weakness on one or both sides of the body (unilateral most common)

Rapid, strong pulse

Sudden weakness or paralysis of face, arm, or leg

Treatment: Do not ignore the signs of a stroke. Call 911 immediately for emergency help or transport immediately to an emergency room. Continually check the persons airway and level of consciousness, as the condition can change rapidly. Give the person 1 to 10 dropperfuls of cayenne tincture orally. Often the stimulation of cayenne if given quickly will pull the person out of danger and improve the recovery. The longer the brain is deprived of blood and oxygen the greater will be the damage. Act quickly. Herbs such as gingko, Motherwort, and Gotu kola are also useful, but none are as dramatic and quick acting as cayenne. Be prepared to administer CPR if necessary.

Long term care is directed towards increasing circulation to the brain, following a health promoting diet, exercising as per doctors recommendations. Do not neglect cleansing the channels of elimination (colon, kidney, lungs, skin and liver).

SWALLOWED OBJECTS

Small, round object (beads, buttons, coins, marbles) swallowed by children usually pass uneventfully through the intestines and are eliminated. Do not give the child cathartics (laxatives) or bulky foods - just the normal diet. If there is pain, or if the child develops a cough, consult your healthcare practitioner.

Sharp or straight objects (bobby pins, open safety pins, bones) are dangerous. Don't panic; consult a doctor. Special instruments may be required to locate and remove the object.

UNCONSCIOUSNESS
Cause Unknown

If you encounter an unconscious person, and the nature of the trouble is unknown: Open the airway (see page 19). If the victim is not breathing or is breathing with great difficulty, apply artificial respiration (see page 18). If his pulse has stopped, begin CPR (see page 24). Check for emergency medical identification, perhaps a card stating that the victim is diabetic (see page 29) or epileptic (see page 31) or some other specific illness. If the victim's face is pale, pulse weak, lower his head slightly. If his lips are blue, check his breathing and pulse. Give one to two droppersful of cayenne tincture then begin artificial respiration or CPR as appropriate. If an unconscious person vomits, to prevent choking turn him on his side if his neck is not broken. Get as full a report as possible as to what happened; ask everyone present.

Have someone call an ambulance. Do not move the victim unless absolutely necessary to prevent further harm. (See "Moving an Injured Person" page 37). Do not disturb or remove an unconscious stranger's personal effects, or anything that may be evidence of a crime or attempted suicide, unless it is essential to save the person's life. Remember: Don't give fluids to an unconscious person.

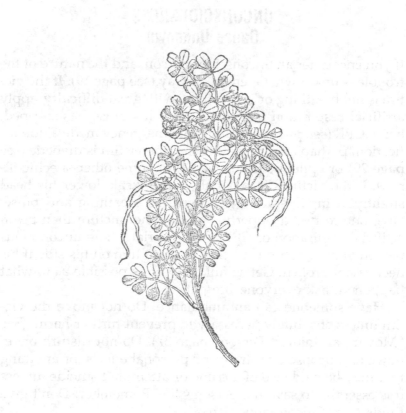

Chapter 3

ABDOMINAL PROBLEMS

ABDOMINAL PROBLEMS

Symptoms	Possible Causes
Nausea or vomiting	See nausea, vomiting, page 64, dehydration, page 148 Medication reaction. Food poisoning, page 157. See Headache, page 115 &/or Head Injury, page 32.

Bowel Movements

Frequent, watery stools	See diarrhea, page 53, food poisoning, page 157 watch for dehydration.
Stools dry and difficult to pass.	Constipation, page 51
Bloody or black, tarry stools.	Ulcers, page 63
Pain during bowel movements; bright red blood on surface of stool or on toilet paper.	Hemorrhoids, page 57

Abdominal Pain

Pain and tenderness in the	Appendicitis, page 48

lower right abdomen with nausea, vomiting, & fever.

Urinary Tract Infections, page 64

Bloating with diarrhea.

Irritable Bowel Syndrome, constipation, or both page 51

Burning or discomfort just below the breastbone.

Ulcers, page 64
Hiatal Hernia, page 60

Pain in the lower abdomen and lower back just before menstrual period.

Menstrual cramps, page142

Urination

Pain or burning on urination

Urinary Tract Infections, page 64

Prostate Problems, page 62

Sexually Transmitted Diseases, page 65

Difficult urination or weak stream (men).

Prostate Problems, page 62

Blood in the urine

Urinary Tract Infections, page 64

Abdominal Lumps or Swelling

Painless lump or swelling in groin that comes & goes

Hernia, page 59

Blow to the stomach; very rigid or distended abdomen

See Blunt Abdominal Wounds, page 48

Watch for Shock

Abdominal organs are either solid or hollow. Solid organs, like the liver and the spleen, when injured, can literally break and bleed internally. Hollow organs such as the intestines can rupture and their contents can drain into the abdominal and pelvic cavities resulting in infection and septicemia (toxicity).

Organ	Type	Quadrant
Liver	Solid	RUQ
Stomach	Hollow	RUQ
Spleen	Solid	LUQ

Pancreas	Solid	LUQ
Intestines (small & large)	Hollow	All Quadrants
Bladder	Hollow	RLQ, LLQ, central
Uterus	Hollow	central
Kidneys	Solid	Flanks

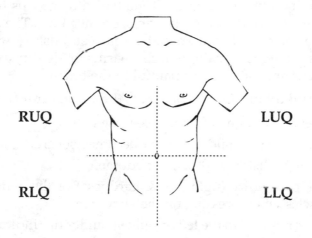

RUQ   LUQ

RLQ   LLQ

ABDOMINAL INJURIES

Penetrating Injuries (Gunshot & Stab Wounds)

Treatment:

1. Call 911 or immediately evacuate the victim.

2. Treat for shock (see page 39).

3. Eviscerated (protruding) bowel should not be placed back into the abdominal cavity. Cover the bowel that is sticking out with sterile dressings and keep them moist with disinfected water at all times. Several more layers of dressings or a towel should be placed over the wound to decrease heat loss.

4. Leave any impaled object in place and stabilize it with bulky dressings or clothing and tape. This will protect it from being jarred and causing more damage.

5. Cayenne pepper is given to prevent shock as well as stop

the bleeding and keep the circulatory system in check. If the persons life is slipping away do not be afraid to give too much cayenne. Lobelia can also be given to help the person relax and ease the pain.

Blunt Abdominal Injuries

A blow to the belly can result in internal organ injuries and bleeding, even though nothing penetrates the skin. Examine the abdomen by pressing on it gently with the tips of your fingers in each of the four quadrants, one at a time. The patient lying on their back with knees bent is best. Push slowly and observe for signs of pain, muscle spasms or rigidity. Normal abdomens are soft and not painful to the touch.

Signs And Symptoms Of Internal Abdominal Injuries:

1. Observe for signs of shock, see page 39;
2. Pain at first is mild and then becomes severe;
3. Bloating (distention) of the abdomen;
4. Pain, or rigidity (tightness & hardness) of the abdominal muscles when pressing on the abdomen;
5. Pain is referred to the left or right shoulder tip (indication of a possible ruptured spleen);
6. Nausea or repetitive vomiting;
7. Bloody urination;
8. Pain in the abdomen on movement;
9. Fever.
   Treatment:
1. Call 911 or evacuate immediately to a medical facility
2. Treat for shock. Anticipate it.
3. Do not allow the patient to eat. If the patient is not vomiting they may have small sips of water.
4. Cayenne tincture taken orally to abate internal bleeding as well as prevent shock. Do not underestimate the power of cayenne pepper in the treatment of acute injuries.

APPENDICITIS

Definition/Diagnosis: Appendicitis is the result of chronic constipation creating an impaction of fecal material and a blockage forming within the appendix. Rarely does appendicitis appear without warning signs of pain and cramping in the lower right region of the abdomen. Treat constipation early with diet and herbs (see "Colon Cleanse" page 254 and The Health Building Diet page 243)

Note: In the event of appendicitis, do not give the person a laxative (herbal or otherwise). Forceful contractions of the bowel caused by the laxative can rupture the appendix. Take the persons temperature. The infection associated with appendicitis will result with a fever. Feel the abdomen while the patient lying down with knees bent thus relaxing the abdominal muscles. If there is any fever, even slight, and if the abdomen feels hard or tense and is sore and painful to the touch, especially on the right lower side, call a doctor at once or take the person to the hospital emergency room. The trouble may be appendicitis.

Other appendicitis symptoms are nausea, vomiting, and persistent pain (lasting over 4 hours). When there is pain in the lower right side of the abdomen, suspect appendicitis until another diagnosis is proved. Meanwhile, if the pain is severe, don't let the person eat or drink anything.

TREATMENT

Mild Attack- This will be recognized as slight aching or pain in the right lower quadrant of the abdomen. Drink 2-4 cups of Red Raspberry leaf tea per day until irritation stops. Follow a mucus-less diet as described in the Health Promoting Diet page 243. Castor oil packs over the area will relax and soften the inflamed tissue (see page 211-212).

Severe Attack- Apply Lobelia Tincture(4 to 6 dropperfuls) and hot Castor oil fomentation (see page 211) over appendix area with knees bent or feet elevated. Caution do not use cold or forceful enemas as they can cause the appendix to rupture. A lukewarm Catnip tea enema can be used to encourage emptying of the rectum and sigmoid colon. You may use a bulb syringe (1 to 3 oz.), which will allow a limited amount of fluid into the colon to help move waste material out. More than anything this rectal injection will stimulate bowel contractions causing a normal bowel movement relieving pressure at the appendix.

Note: never use a full enema on a person with suspected

appendicitis. Then apply alternating hot and cold packs over the area until attack is over. Ten minutes hot, ten minutes cold. Use "direction of energy" treatments as described on page 263. Once out of crisis, use a castor oil pack over the area for 1 to 2 hours kept warm with a hot water bottle. Use just enough Colon Cleanse to insure proper bowel movement beginning a couple days after the attack has subsided.

APPETITE, loss of

Poor appetite is not a disorder in itself, but usually a symptom of some other problem. Emotional factors such as depression, illness or stress and trauma can reduce ones appetite. Substance addiction such as alcohol or tobacco use or poisoning with heavy metals can be the cause.

Herbal appetite stimulants such as Yarrow, catnip, fennel seed, ginger root, ginseng, papaya leaves or peppermint tea or tincture in hot water 2 times daily can be very effective. Learn and correct the underlying cause.

COLIC

Colon Cleanse to insure 2-3 bowel movements per day. Ginger tea, 1 cup per day. For small infants use catnip tea or Catnip/Fennel Tincture or Glycerite. Adults can make a Slippery Elm gruel (Add water to Slippery Elm to make a paste. Then add more water for gruel-like consistency - it's kind of slimy but it really works). Colitis Formula, take 3-5 capsules or as needed. The use of a catnip enema and a castor oil fomentation over the abdomen kept warm with a hot water bottle will soothe things down. Digestive enzymes are also highly recommended.

COLITIS/IRRITABLE BOWEL SYNDROME

Definition/Diagnosis: Sharp abdominal pains and cramping can be debilitating. Typically a person suffering from colitis will have a history and will be familiar with what is going on. There are two concerns here. Pain relief and preventing dehydration. The irritable bowel can have as many as 50 burning bowel movements in a day. This condition is often emotionally triggered.

Treatment: Apply a hot water bottle to the abdomen. Drink a carminative tea such as chamomile, catnip or fennel. Slippery elm gruel is soothing. For acute episodes an enema of aloe vera is very soothing, cooling and healing. Take Colitis Formula (see page 222) on a regular basis and follow the Health Promoting Diet. Dietary , food allergy and stress issues need to be corrected. Food allergies can play a major role is colitis and irritable bowel. This requires come detective work or visiting someone trained in BioSET or muscle testing techniques for identifying and eliminating allergies.

CONSTIPATION (see Colon Cleanse page 254)

Definition/Diagnosis: Signs of an Unclean Colon - Gas, flatulence, foul breath, bad body odor, acne, digestive problems, infections of the kidney, prostate, bladder, liver and / or gallbladder, excess mucus in the head, lungs, and /or throat, chronic sickness with all types of disorders. Begin to be concerned if the person hasn't had a bowel movement for 3 days. If the five day mark is approaching, they have become a patient and herbal laxatives are necessary. Don't let it get this far. Our bowels should be moving 2 to 3 times daily.

Prevention: Prevention is the best medicine. Eat a proper diet. - predominantly whole grains with the addition of fresh or frozen fruits and vegetables. Chew your food thoroughly. Eat slowly. Avoid red meat and poultry. Eat fish a couple times per week. Drink plenty of water. Eating meals that contain both hot and cold foods get the digestive juices flowing and help the bowels to move. Dehydration is probably the most common cause of constipation. Exercise daily. Exercise will help to strengthen and tone the digestive tract. Do not resist "the call". Go to the bathroom when you need to. Tobacco and caffeine have a paralyzing effect on the colon and encourage constipation. Coffee also destroys the "friendly bacteria" in the large intestine. Alcohol tends to produce constipation and increased intestinal mucus. Juices such as prune juice are often beneficial to help the lower bowel. Do not use a laxative either medicinal or herbal. Rather use an herbal bowel tonic, such as Colon Cleanse (see page 222). Periodic cleansing of your colon with Colon Detox (see page 223) is another way to insure good colon health.

Treatment: The object is to catch constipation early enough that you do not have to undergo heroic efforts. Begin with a good herbal laxative (Colon Cleanse, page 222) and drinking plenty of water or herbal tea. Often a change in the diet is enough. Rarely are enemas necessary and even less likely is the use of a latex glove to manually remove the impacted feces. When the colon is cleansed, many different disorders and ailments clear up on their own as the body can begin functioning the way it was designed to.

If there is a fever involved drink plenty of yarrow, peppermint, red raspberry leaf or catnip tea (8 to 16 cups in 24 hours). Take Colon Cleanse (see page 256) beginning with one capsule per day (take with a meal) and increasing the dosage each day until you are having 2-3 bowel movements daily. Using Colon Detox (see page 257) can cleanse the bowel of impurities and toxicity. A very good bowel cleansing program can be found using Colon Detox in conjunction with Colon Cleanse.

CRAMPS

Definition/Diagnosis: A cramp is a muscle screaming for help. The pain is from a lack of oxygen getting to the muscle cells. As the muscle fibers tighten and cramp, they constrict the arteries and capillaries that provide their blood circulation. Over-stretching, blunt trauma or metabolic conditions, such as dehydration, can cause muscle cramps.

Treatment: The object in treating is to restore the circulation to the affected area. Generally 1 to 2 dropperfuls of lobelia tincture works very well. Lobelia is a very powerful relaxant.

Menstrual:	1-2 dropperfuls of Female Balancing Formula 3 times daily. Pain formula as needed. Massage cinnamon leaf essential oil to abdomen. Hot water bottle over uterus with ice pack on forehead or back of neck.
Muscle:	Lobelia tincture massaged into muscle spasm. Deep Heat oil massaged into

	muscle spasm.
Stomach:	Technically different than a cramp involving a muscle but the principle still applies. Soothe and relax the area allowing better flow and circulation. Ginger root tea, Peppermint tea, Fennel tea, or Cinnamon tea - 2 cups a day as needed.

DIARRHEA

Definition/Diagnosis: The definition of diarrhea is having 2 to 3 times the number of bowel movements that are customary for an individual. These stools can be either soft (meaning they hold shape) or watery (meaning they can be poured). By definition, in order to have the diagnosis of diarrhea, one should have at least one of these other symptoms; fever chills, abdominal cramps, nausea, or vomiting. Diarrhea is generally self-limiting, lasting 2 to 3 days. An acute onset of watery diarrhea usually means that E. coli or shigellosis is the cause. Symptoms of bloody diarrhea or mucous in the stools are frequently seen with an infection of Shigella, Campylobacter, or Salmonella. The presence of chronic diarrhea with malabsorbtion and gas indicates that Giardia may be present.

The major concern with diarrhea is the amount of fluid lost or the dehydration that results. The degree of dehydration can be estimated from certain signs and symptoms:

Mild Dehydration (3-5% weight loss) is characterized by thirst, tacky mucous around lips and mouth, normal pulse, and dark urine.

Moderate Dehydration (5-10% weight loss) is characterized by thirst, dry mucous membranes (lips and mouth), sunken eyes, only a small volume of dark urine, and a rapid, weak pulse.

Severe Dehydration (over 10% weight loss) is characterized by drowsiness, lethargy, very dry mucous membranes, sunken eyes, no urine production, no tears, and shock. The pulse with be rapid, thready or difficult to feel.

Treatment:

1. Replace Fluid and Electrolytes. Oral rehydration with water and electrolytes (body salts and minerals) is the most important treatment for diarrhea illnesses. The fluids and electrolytes that are lost from dehydration can become fatal. The body has the ability to absorb water and electrolytes given orally, even during severe bouts of diarrhea. The fluid expelled with diarrhea contain sodium chloride (salt), potassium and bicarbonate, so simply drinking plain water is not an adequate replacement. Most sports drinks should not be used because they are too high in sugars and do not have the proper electrolyte balance. Gatorade can be used if diluted to half strength with water.

   Oral Rehydration Solution (ORS)
   1 teaspoon of salt (sea salt is preferred)
   4 teaspoons of cream of tartar (potassium bicarbonate)
   1/2 teaspoon baking soda
   4 Tablespoons of sugar
   1 quart (or liter) of water
   Or
   8 oz. fruit juice with 1/2 tsp. honey and a pinch of salt followed by 8 oz. water with 1/2 tsp. of baking soda.

2. Mildly or moderately dehydrated adults should drink between 4 to 6 quarts (or liters) of ORS (Oral Rehydration Solution) in the first four to six hours. Children can be given eight ounces of ORS every hour. Severe dehydration usually requires fluids to be given intravenously.

3. Rice, bananas and potatoes are good to be eaten to supplement rehydration. Fats, dairy products, caffeine, and alcohol should be strictly avoided. Avoid drinking full strength juices. Juices usually have 3 to 5 times the amount of sugar and can make diarrhea worse.

4. Using Colon Detox (page 223) can help to trap and pull toxins from the bowel and slow down motility. This remedy will also help with the gas and cramping. Take one heaping teaspoon of Colon Detox powder mixed with water every hour until diarrhea stops. Slippery Elm gruel

can also be used (2 tsp. slippery elm to 6 oz. liquid) to slow down motility. Chamomile tea or comfrey and catnip combined in a tea are useful. Drink 2 to 3 cups daily. Plantain in a tea or tincture can be used orally. For severe cases of diarrhea catnip tea can be used in an enema to calm the bowel down as well as help with rehydration.

5. If fever is present, treat as you would an infection with immune boosting herbs (echinacea, garlic, Goldenseal, cat's claw, Pau d' Arco, Immune Boost (page 230), and Anti-Plague Syrup (page 219).

DIARRHEA - Traveler's Diarrhea

Definition/Diagnosis: This refers to diarrhea that occurs in the context of foreign as well as some domestic travel. It usually occurs when people visit underdeveloped or third-world countries. Symptoms usually begin abruptly two or three days into the trip. The diarrhea can be watery or soft, and there can be cramping, nausea, vomiting, fatigue and fever.

Treatment: Treat as you would diarrhea with an emphasis on herbal treatments for fever and parasites. Use herbal parasite formula and eat pumpkin seeds. See parasites, page 172.

Prevention: Traveler's diarrhea is caused by bacteria and afflicts almost 50% of visitors to underdeveloped countries. It is acquired through the ingestion of contaminated food or water. Watching what you eat and drink may help but does not guarantee that you will not get sick. A person traveling should avoid drinking untreated tape water or drinks with ice cubes. Bottled and carbonated drinks are generally safe. Custards, salads, salsas, and reheated food, milk fruits and vegetables should be avoided. Be careful of any fresh or unprocessed foods. Peel all fresh fruits and vegetables. Often, in countries lacking refrigeration, fruits and vegetables are 'refreshened' on the way to market by sprinkling these foods with water from the roadside drainage ditches. The use of human fertilizer makes this water very contaminated. Fruits and vegetables sold by their weight are often injected with "water" to increase their weight and resale value. Washing the produce thoroughly is not effective in this case. Disinfect your tap water even before brushing your teeth.

Less severe cases are often experienced traveling domestically simply due to a change in the food and water that your body have become accustomed to. Use the same steps above is these cases too.

Colloidal silver (40 ppm) 1 to 2 tsp. three times daily can be taken prophylactically.

FLATULENCE (Gas, stomach and bowels)

Definition/Diagnosis: When food is poorly digested it can ferment and become sour causing gas anywhere along the digestive tract. This symptom can be painful, smelly and embarrassing. Often the cause is as simple as eating too fast, overeating or eating unhealthy (junk) foods.

Treatment: For gas use either digestive enzymes or herbal digestive aids, such as fennel, cinnamon, peppermint, or chlorophyll. Wild Yam or celery seed tea (made into an infusion or decoction) are effective. Goldenseal with myrrh (equal parts) is an excellent stomach tonic. Eliminate carbonated drinks and foods that cause gas.

Use Colon Cleanse as directed. Ginger tea 1-2 cups per day. Fennel Tea 1-2 cups per day. Use a hot water bottle for gas pains and or cramping.

GALLBLADDER (Complaints)

Definition/Diagnosis: The gallbladder is a small pouch shaped organ located under the liver. It stores and concentrates bile that is secreted by the liver during digestion to help break up or digest fat in the diet. If the gallbladder becomes inflamed it cause severe pain in the upper right abdomen. Often gallbladder pain is referred to the right scapula and shoulder. Sometimes cholesterol crystallizes and combines with bile creating gallstones. If the stones block the bile duct pain, nausea and vomiting may occur. Often symptoms are triggered by eating fatty foods.

Treatment for inflammation and pain:

1. Stop eating for a couple of days.
2. Drink only distilled water with lemon.
3. Drink as much pure apple juice as possible for the next five days.

4. To relieve pain, use a hot castor oil pack over the gallbladder. Heat castor oil in a pan (don't boil). Dip a piece of flannel or other white cotton material and saturate with the castor oil. Apply over the liver/gallbladder area. It should be warm, but not too hot. Cover with a large piece of plastic then place a hot water bottle over the area to keep it warm. Keep warm for 1-1/2 to 2 hours or as needed. You may store the used castor oil pack in plastic or a zip lock for up to 20 uses.

5. Use a coffee enema to cleanse the liver and gallbladder.

6. Avoid spicy foods, animal foods, fatty foods and oils. Eat a 75% raw foods diet.

7. Liver-Gallbladder Flush as described on pages 257-258.

8. Colon Cleanse as needed for 2-3 normal bowel movements daily.

GASTRITIS and HEARTBURN

Definition/Diagnosis: A burning sensation in the middle of the upper part of the abdomen (mid-epigastric is most likely gastritis or heartburn. Often associated with over-eating or eating just before bedtime. Advertisers have spent millions to get you to spell "relief" there way and chew antacid products. Chronic use of antacids can cause malabsorbtion problems. Often nausea will accompany this heartburn. Gastritis can develop into an ulcer if left untreated.

Treatment: Eat slowly. Chew your food thoroughly. Set your fork down between bites. To increase hydrochloric acid function and digestion, take Apple Cider Vinegar and Honey (mixed 50/50). 2 Tbs. in water or juice 3 times daily. This will help to restore normal HCl (hydrochloric acid) secretions. Slippery elm gruel (2 Tbs. to 1 cup water) is soothing and effective in relieving stomach pain. Carminative herbs, such as peppermint, cinnamon and licorice will promote digestion and relieve pain. Instead of using antacids, switch to something that will promote digestion function such as Altoids™ or digestive enzymes.

HEMORRHOIDS (Piles)

Definition/Diagnosis: Hemorrhoids, also called piles, is a painful swollen cluster of varicose veins around the rectum. External hemorrhoids are small, rounded purplish masses which become enlarged when straining on the stool. Unless a blood clot forms in them, they are soft and tender. When clots form, they become excruciatingly painful. Hemorrhoids are the most common cause of rectal bleeding, with the blood also appearing on the toilet paper. It often takes about five days for the clots to absorb thus decreasing pain and allowing the mass to regress. Rectal skin tags can be a result of chronic hemorrhoids.

Treatment: There are a variety of natural treatments that are effective in treating and reducing hemorrhoids.

1. Moist heat gives the most effective relief during an acute flair up. Heat a cloth in water and apply it for 15 minutes, 4 times daily.

2. Avoid any constipation by taking Colon Cleanse (page 222), drinking adequate amounts of water (8 - 10 cups daily) and following a health promoting diet (page 243).

3. Cayenne pepper taken orally increases the circulation and will help to get rid of stagnant blood causing painful hemorrhoids. Start with 1/4 tsp. of cayenne powder in juice or water and work up to 1 to 3 tsp. of cayenne 3 times daily. Cayenne oil or deep heat oil or ointment (page 225) can be rubbed directly into the hemorrhoidal tissue. This will cause the swelling to shrink down and eventually be eliminated. To make your own cayenne oil; use 5 Tbs. of powdered cayenne - the hotter the better - to 20 ounces of olive or Jojoba oil, shake daily for 14 days, then strain.

4. A raw peeled potato suppository can offer great relief. Cut the potato to the size of a French fry. Insert into rectum and hold for several hours or until next bowel movement.

5. CTR Ointment applied topically over affected area is soothing and helpful.

6. Witch Hazel made into a tea or an over-the-counter preparation is effective used topically because of its astringent properties.

7. Other astringent herbs such as Oak bark or gall are effective in reducing the swelling (apply topically). Oak bark powder can be mixed with glycerin and used as a suppository.

8. Dietary changes are a must for the long term management of hemorrhoids. Eat a high fiber, plant based diet. Avoid consti-

pating foods such as meat, cheese, and dairy products.

HERNIA

Definition/Diagnosis: A hernia occurs when there is a weakening and separation of muscles in the abdominal wall allowing the pressure of the gut (the intestines) against the opening or muscle separation to push through. Healing to the point of complete repair without surgical intervention is unlikely. The most common hernia in a male is an inguinal hernia, which is an out-pouching of the intestines through a weak area located above and on either side of the penis. Pushing up into the abdominal wall through the scrotum will find this, often causing great discomfort.

Hernias can also occur in the abdominal wall near the umbilicus (belly button). A hernia can occur while straining (lifting, coughing, sneezing, etc.). There is typically a sharp pain at the location of the hernia and the person will note a bulge. This bulge may disappear when the patient lies on their back and relaxes. If the intestine in the hernia is squeezed by the abdominal wall to the point that the blood supply is cut off, the hernia is termed a "strangulated" hernia. This is a medical emergency, as the loop of gut in the hernia will die, turn gangrenous, and lead to a generalized abdominal infection. This condition is much worse than appendicitis and death will result if not treated surgically.

A hernia that fails to reduce, or disappear when the person relaxes on their back is considered "incarcerated". While this may turn into an emergency, it is not one at that point. Most hernias' caused by straining in adults will not strangulate. Further straining should be avoided. If lifting or physically straining and working is necessary, or while coughing and sneezing, the person should protect himself from further tissue damage by pressing against the area with one hand, thus holding the hernia in.

Treatment: CTR ointment applied at night over the affected area. Hernias should be treated as an injury and can potentially be very dangerous and often require surgical repair. An evaluation by a health care provider is recommended. Active hernias generally will not respond to herbal packs, poultices or fomentations.

HIATAL HERNIA (see also indigestion)

Definition/Diagnosis: This condition is often seen as heartburn or reflux esophagitis. While not a first aid emergency, it can cause considerable discomfort. The habitual or daily use of antacids may afford very temporary relief, but will worsen the condition in the long run.

Treatment: Eat small meals based on "the health promoting diet", see page 243. Traction the stomach downward. This very effective maneuver can work tremendously. The patient stands leaning their back to the wall. Have the patient take a deep breath and as they exhale push with fingertips inward at the epigastric area (where the ribs come together above the abdomen in the midline) and traction downward. With each exhalation push a little deeper and traction down a little harder. This will be a little uncomfortable for the patient. They can thank you afterwards. Digestive herbs, such as peppermint, licorice root, fennel, catnip, cinnamon, etc. should also be used on a regular basis. Eat slowly and chew your food thoroughly (thoroughly means to chew your food until it is the consistency of applesauce). And most especially, DO NOT OVEREAT.

INDIGESTION

Definition/Diagnosis: As with any condition, always attempt to determine the cause, then treat accordingly. Hallmarked by burning in the back of the throat and may be accompanied by bloating, gas, and stomach cramping. Indigestion is common in those who typically are aware they already suffer from it. If indigestion is bran new to the person, explore other causative factors as well as simple indigestion. Chewing antacids is not the solution even though they are highly promoted through advertising. An antacid does neutralize the acid in the stomach, however in so doing it ceases digestion and creates more chronic problems. You do much better to stimulate the digestive process rather than paralyze it.

Treatment: Use just about any of the carminative herbs. These herbs are the ones that taste good such as Ginger, Peppermint, Licorice root, Fennel, or Cinnamon. Take as a tincture or make into a tea. Nettle Tincture - 1-2 dropperfuls 3 times daily.

The essential oil of these carminative herbs (one drop on

the tongue) is also effective. Cramp bark and Wild Yam tinctures can also be effectively used. Massaging lobelia tincture over the stomach (more specifically the epigastric area - where the lower rib cage meets in the center) can offer immediate relief. Also take 2 to 3 drops of lobelia orally. Take the herbs before meals if you're prone to indigestion. Do no overeat - this is probably the biggest cause of indigestion. USe enzymes!

KIDNEY INFECTIONS (Pyelonephritis)

Definition/Diagnosis: An infection that settles in the kidneys usually begins in the bladder. Often a kidney infection will produce lower back pain that can be mistaken for a back injury.

Treatment: Treat as you would a urinary tract infection (see page 64) with emphasis on using the immune building herbs (garlic, echinacea, etc.).

KIDNEY STONES

Definition/Diagnosis: Kidney stones are hard deposits that develop in the urinary tract and produce extreme pain that is often felt in the back. The stones range in size from a grain of sand to a marble and are three times more common in men than women. They typically occur in middle age (40 to 60). Dehydration and a diet high in protein or calcium are predisposing factors. Often the first symptom is very sharp and severe pain which is often debilitating. The pain usually starts in the flank area or on one side of the back radiating into the abdomen or groin. The person can often be seen, with knees drawn up, rolling from one side to the other trying to find a comfortable position. With appendicitis or other abdominal infection, the victim will try to lie still because movement increases the pain. Not so with kidney stones. Other symptoms may include nausea, vomiting, an urge to urinate, and blood in the urine.

Treatment:

1. Drink plenty of fluids - at least one gallon in 24 hours. The more the better. Drink water, herb tea or fresh apple juice. No coffee, alcohol, soda pop or caffeine in any form.
2. Stone Dissolve Tea is best. This is made with equal parts Gravel root, Hydrangea root, Marshmallow root and Rose hips. Drink one gallon of this tea per day.

3. Kidney-Bladder Tea also works very well and should be used for maintenance. Drinking this tea will help to dissolve, flush out and prevent new stones from forming.

The Kidney-Bladder Flush as described on page 259 is useful both for prevention as well as treatment.

Herbal pain formula can be used hourly or as needed. Most kidney stones will pass on their own. (see page 233)

Occasionally, kidney stones can lead to infection and can damage the kidneys. Rarely do they require surgical removal. Dissolving them Herbally, really is the way to go.

PROSTATE (Complaints)

Definition/Diagnosis: The prostate is a walnut sized male sex gland the encircles the urinary outlet (the urethra). It can become swollen constricting the urine flow. When enlarged the bladder may not be able to be completely emptied. This can result in bladder and kidney infections.

Treatment: Immediate treatment is the Kidney-Bladder Formula, see page 230. Diuretic herbs and urinary tonics such as juniper berries, parsley, uva ursi, and corn silk are beneficial. Juniper berries are a disinfectant as well as a diuretic.

Use Prostate Plus Formula (Saw Palmetto & Pygeum bark) as directed, drink copious amounts of watermelon juice. Drink kidney-bladder tea. Take Colon Cleanse as needed. All dairy products with the exception of yogurt must be eliminated from the diet as well as meat (beef, chicken, turkey, pork, etc.). Cold water fish eaten 2 to 3 times per week is acceptable.

TESTICLE - Painful

Definition/Diagnosis: Spontaneous swelling of the scrotum with enlargement of a testicle can be due to an infection of the testicle (orchitis) or more commonly an infection of the sperm collecting duct called the epididymis (epididymitis).

Treatment: If the pain is severe, lie the person on his back with a cloth draped over both thighs and looping under the scrotum forming a sling or cradle on which the scrotum may rest. Ice packs or a towel soaked in cold water or an herbal tea made with 3 parts mullein and 1 part lobelia will be soothing. Keep the area moist by continuing to add the mullein/lobelia tea. In addition drink 3 to 6 cups of Mullein/Lobelia tea daily.

Begin the use of Immune Boost hourly (1-2 dropperfuls) orally. Diet should consist of fresh raw fruits and vegetables. No mucus producing foods such as dairy and meats should be eaten.

The problem may not be due to an infection. It is possible for the testicle to become twisted, due to a slight congenital defect, resulting in severe pain. This is called "testicular torsion" and can be a surgical emergency. Testicular torsion can be very difficult to distinguish from orchitis. Since the testicle always seems to rotate "inward" often immediate relief can be found by rotating the testicle "outward". If the problem is not a rotated testicle, no harm will be done by this maneuver. But if it is you will have saved yourself a trip to the emergency room. A person with severe testicular pain needs immediate attention. An unreduced testicular torsion can become gangrenous with a life threatening infection resulting.

ULCERS - stomach/duodenal

Definition/Diagnosis: Increased stomach acid (usually associated with gastritis) can lead to stomach or duodenal ulcers. A bacterial infection has also been implicated as a causative factor. Pain will be burning and often associated with eating and/or stress. Pain within a half hour after eating is associated with duodenal ulcers. An old herbal formula (Robert's Formula) has been effectively used for the treatment of digestive tract also. Much of its' success may be because it uses antibacterial herbs as well as stomach herbs.

Treatment:

1. Often a glass a cold water alone with provide quick relief.

2. Cayenne Tincture(30 drops) or 1/2 teaspoon powder in water 2 times daily is effective . Cayenne works very fast in providing relief. Cayenne will feed the mucus membranes of the digestive tract restoring the Iron and Calcium which may have been lost.

3. Drink fresh Cabbage Juice.

4. Eat Slippery Elm gruel to soothe stomach.

5. Several scientific studies have demonstrated that licorice root is more effective than Tagamet and Zantac in heal-

ing peptic ulcers and licorice root can also prevent reoccurrence.

URINARY TRACT INFECTIONS (UTI's) - see also cystitis pg. 133

Definition/Diagnosis: Women tend to be more susceptible than men which can stem from poor or improper personal hygiene. Too little fluid intake with a high protein diet will change the pH, making UTI's more likely. Burning pain with urination are the hallmark of a urinary tract infection. The infection is typically from the bladder (cystitis), but could be from the kidneys or ureters (the tubes from the kidneys to the bladder) as well. If not treated quickly and completely a UTI can lead to serious kidney damage.

Treatment: Kidney-Bladder formula (page 230) 1 dropperful in Kidney-Bladder Tea - 3 to 16 cups per day depending on severity. The more tea the better. Cranberry juice is often used. Cranberry juice does not directly fight the infection, rather it make the walls of bladder slippery so that the bacteria/ virus etc. cannot adhere themselves. It is vitally important that plenty of fluid are consumed. Strive for a full gallon of herbal tea in a 24 hour period. The herbal combination above works wonders, even on bladder infections that have survived several rounds of antibiotics. Resolution of symptoms is usually within 8 to 12 hours. However continue drinking the Kidney-Bladder tea and associated herbs for several days just to be sure. Virulent and persistent infections rarely return after being treated with these herbs. Immune Boost or echinacea should also be used to strengthen the immune system to fight any infection.

VOMITING

Definition/Diagnosis: Nausea and vomiting are often caused by infections such as gastroenteritis. Many times these are viral so that antibiotic therapy will have no positive effect. These infections may be associated with diarrhea (see page 53) and usually resolve on their own in 24 to 48 hours. If a fever persists for more than 12 hours, treat as you would an infectious illness.

The big question should always be WHY. Vomiting is often an important aspect of the body's defense mechanism. It is the quickest most efficient way to remove the contents of the stomach and even the upper portion of the small intestines (duodenum). Remember to treat the cause. If vomiting is due to food or chemical poisoning, refer to that section (page 157).

To Stop: 2-6 drops of Lobelia Tincture or 1-2 cups Ginger tea. Red Raspberry tea can also calm the stomach.

To Induce: 1 tsp. to 1 Tbs. Lobelia Tincture to rid stomach of toxins. Tickling the back of the throat is probably the quickest way to induce vomiting. Check the poisoning section for possible contraindications.

SEXUALLY TRANSMITTED DISEASES

It is beyond the scope of this book to discuss in any length sexually transmitted or venereal diseases. Do not overlook the possibility of a STD with genital and/or urinary complaints. If left untreated many of these diseases can cause serious permanent harm and even death. See your medical doctor for proper diagnosis and treatment.

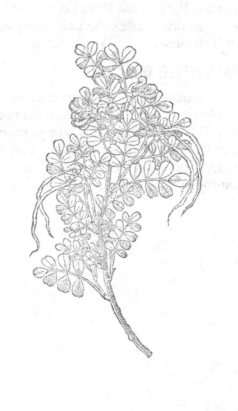

Chapter 4

BONE, MUSCLE & JOINT PROBLEMS

ARTHRITIS

Arthritis is the inflammation of one or more joints. It is characterized by pain, swelling, stiffness and eventually deformity and a reduced normal range of motion. Deep Heat oil or ointment massaged in afflicted area, CTR ointment and syrup, Apple Cider Vinegar/Honey, and **Arthritis Formula** all are helpful (see page 222). A strict vegetarian/vegan diet can provide the most long term benefits.

BRUISES AND CONTUSIONS

Immediately after the injury, place an insulated ice bag or cold compress (a small towel soaked in ice water and wrung out) over the bruise. This should reduce the pain and swelling. If the pain persists, or if vision is impaired (as with black eye(s), take the patient to their healthcare provider. Use alternating hot/cold hydrotherapy (see appendix, page 260), afterwards apply Deep Heat Formula (see page 226) then CTR Ointment (see page 224). Take CTR Syrup (see page 224) 2-3 times per day, 1 teaspoon.

ORTHOPEDIC INJURIES (In General)

Orthopedics include injuries of the bones, joints and muscles, their function and their disorders.

General Treatment: First stabilize the injured area whether there is a fracture, dislocation, sprain or strain. The initial treatment for these injuries once stabilized is to use ice to control the inflammation. Use an ice pack 10 to 20 minutes every waking hour for at least the first two days. After that you can begin using alternating hot and cold therapy as described in "Healing Soft Tissue Injuries" page 260. Use herbs to help control pain (see page 233). Complete Tissue Repair Ointment and Syrup (see page 224) are used to provide the body with the nutritional building blocks to speed the healing. Lather the ointment generously over the wound site twice daily. Use the CTR syrup or comfrey tea three times daily (1 tsp. to 1 Tbs.) Comfrey is the principle ingredient that will knit bone and tissue back together. Drink fresh carrot juice 4 to 8 cups daily. Hot fomentations of poultices of comfrey may be used. Use an herbal pain formula (see page 260) (1-4 dropperfuls) as needed (hourly at first).

MUSCLE PAIN - No Acute Injury

Definition/Diagnosis: Muscle aches can arise from chronic inflammatory disorders such as Lupus or Fibromyalgia. Muscle pain that is non-traumatic but more acute (onset is new) in the absence of trauma or injury could be due to overuse (exercise) or possibly infection. When muscles ache and there is a fever present, suspect an infectious origin of the problem. In this case it is best to treat with immune enhancing herbs and procedures such as the cold sheet treatment (see page 248). Check the body for ticks (the insect, not a twitching muscle), as Lyme disease can be a cause for sore muscles. Lyme disease is caused from bites of infected ticks.

Conditions such as heat stress, heavy exertion causing sweating, diarrhea, vomiting, or the use of diuretics (herbal diuretics included) causing increased urine output, can cause muscles to cramp due to a decrease in electrolytes. Replace the fluids if this is the cause. Use 10 to 15 grams of salt with 2 quarts of water. The weight of a nickel is 5 grams, use this as a guide to estimate (i.e. 2-3 nickels worth).

Overuse syndromes cause pain in muscles that are more than just a mild ache you feel after working out too hard. While it is possible to suddenly tear muscles with sudden movements, significant pain that begins gradually or after exercise is over, can represent pain caused by tendonitis, bursitis, or significant inflammation of the muscle. Treat each of these with alternating hot/cold therapy (see page 260) with the use of Deep Heat Ointment or oil. Herbal Pain Formula can calm spasming muscles and provide pain relief.

STRAIN - MUSCLE PAIN - Acute Injury

Definition/Diagnosis: When muscle pain occurs immediately after a significant muscle injury, the cause is either a strain(tearing of muscle fibers) or contusion (an internal bruise to the muscle).

Treatment: Remember the acronym RICE: Rest, Ice, Compress, Elevate. Use of an elastic or Ace bandage, and ice pack or cold stream of water, elevation of a limb and resting should be adhered to for the first 24 to 48 hours. After this time alternating hot and cold water or compresses can be introduced. (See page 260). The most important thing you can do initially after the injury is use ice or cold water . **Caution: Do not freeze the injury.** Generally 10 to 20 minutes each hour is sufficient.

Contusions cause bleeding into the surrounding muscle tissue because of the tearing and rupturing of small blood vessels. RICE will minimize the bleeding and keep the swelling to a minimum. Muscular strains result in either microscopic muscle fiber tears or massive muscle tears. Strains are graded from I to IV. Grade I is a microscopic tear. Grade II and III are partial tears of the muscle mass. Grade IV is a total tearing of the muscle, which usually requires surgical repair. A Grade IV tear will be accompanied by the balling up or bulging of the muscle into a knot. It will look and feel like it knotted up and has become detached. This may not become apparent for several days. Once the pain is gone, there will be continued swelling, even after several weeks have passed. There will be major swelling in both a Grade III and Grade IV tear (strain). A Grade IV strain is not a surgical emergency and can be safely done 4 to 6 weeks after the injury.

JOINT PAIN - No Acute Injury
Arthritis, Bursitis, Tendonitis

Definition/Diagnosis: Pain in a joint or joints in the absence of injury is generally due to arthritis, tendonitis or bursitis. If the person doesn't have a history of trauma, arthritis, tendonitis or bursitis are the more likely diagnoses. The most common reason for tendon or joint inflammation is overuse of the joint. Tendonitis commonly occurs in the Achilles tendon (Achilles tendonitis), the lateral elbow (lateral epicondylitis), in the thumb, wrist, shoulder or just about any tendon in the body that can be over used. Joints can also become inflamed with repetitious activity or pressure over the joint. Shoulder bursitis is very common with repetitious arm movements.

Treatment: Avoid the activity or movement which has caused the injury. This can be difficult when the repetitious movement is required for employment, however, often one can learn to use the other limb or an alternative way to perform the task. Often incorrect posture for the task is the cause of the injury. Alternating Hot and Cold Hydrotherapy (see page 260) with the use of Deep Heat Ointment or Oil should be used (see page 225).

Herbal pain support should be used as necessary. Splinting the area may be useful. However, avoid splinting for longer than 2 weeks as scar tissue and adhesions will form within the muscles result in a decrease or loss of function, particularly with the shoulder.

SPRAIN - JOINT PAIN - Acute Injury

Definition/Diagnosis: Unusual stress across a joint can result in damage to the supporting ligaments of that joint. Most often the ligaments (ligaments connect bone to bone, tendons connect muscle to bone), are stretched and micro-tearing occurs. In severe cases ligaments are ruptured, cartilage can tear and even bones can fracture. These severe injuries can require surgical repair. It is best done immediately, but can safely be delayed 2 to 3 months. If a fracture enters the joint space, it can result in long term pain and "post-traumatic arthritis". Cartilage is very difficult to heal and without aggressive herbal treatment (hot/cold hydrotherapy, CTR ointment & syrup, and comfrey compresses), a cartilage tear may require surgical repair. In the event of a sprained ankle, splint the ankle with the boot or shoe on until you are able to get to a place for rest and treatment. Once the boot is off, you may not be able to get it back on due to the swelling.

Treatment: RICE (Rest, Ice, Compress, Elevate) immediately. Apply cold for the first two days as much as possible. After this 48 hours, begin hot/cold hydrotherapy (see page 260). Keep the injured joint elevated above the heart level and keep wrapped with an elastic bandage. Before applying the bandage, coat the joint thickly with Complete Tissue Repair Ointment. Clear plastic wrap may be placed directly against the skin to hold the ointment next to the skin. The plastic wrap will help to keep things neater as well as prevent absorption into the ace or elastic bandage. The elastic bandage should provide the patient with moderate support and immobility. If the wrapping is too tight it may cut off the circulation. Orthopedic padding such as that which is used during the casting of a fractured limb can offer protection if swelling is expected. Use herbs for pain as necessary.

Use crutches or other supports to take the weight and stress off the injured joint. If use, movement or weight bearing causes pain, then you can assume you are putting strain on the joint and can be causing further damage or at least stirring up the inflammation and preventing or slowing the healing process. On the other hand, if use, movement or weight bearing is not painful then you are not causing additional damage even though there may still be swelling. Listen to your body and use your common sense. The more diligent you are taking care of an injury early on then the better will be the long term prognosis.

BROKEN BONES

Keep the broken bone ends and adjacent joints from moving. Maintain the victim's body temperature and, if necessary, treat for shock (see page 39). If a broken bone protrudes through the skin and there is severe bleeding, stop the bleeding (see page 14), but do not attempt to push the bone back into place. Also make no attempt to clean the wound. Call for emergency medical assistance at once.

Don't move the person if the break is in the back, neck, pelvis or skull. (See "Broken Neck or Back," page 76, and "Head Injury", page 32). If the victim of a less serious fracture must he moved to receive medical aid, immobilize the fracture with splints to prevent further damage. (Do not assume that no bones are broken merely because the victim is able to move the injured limb or joint.)

For splints, use anything that will keep the broken bones from moving - newspaper, magazines, broomsticks or boards for arms or legs. Make the splints long enough to reach beyond the joints above and below the break.

In automobile accidents, splint a fractured leg, if possible, before moving the victim from the car. Place cloth padding between the legs. Then, using bandages or other material, tie the injured leg to the uninjured leg above and below the fracture site, and immobilize it as much as possible by using an improvised short splint.

Arm or leg splinting is done merely to immobilize the break. Leave bonesetting to the doctor and splint the limb in the position in which you find it.

If it is impossible to apply a splint without straightening the limb, support it with a hand on either side of the break while someone gently eases it into a position that is as close to natural as possible. Pad improvised splints with cotton or clean rags and tie them snugly (but not too tight) in place with bandages, belts, neckties or strips of clothing. The pulses distal (downstream) from the splinting should be checked before and after you splint. If you find that a pulse is lost or diminished after you splint, your splint in not right. Circulation must remain good. Take off the splint and re-do it.

Once the fracture has been stabilized assist the healing process through the use of herbal therapy.

Herbally: Apply CTR ointment over affected area as you are able. More importantly, take CTR Syrup 3-5 times daily.

Drinking comfrey leaf or root tea - 3 to 6 cups per day is advisable. A comfrey leaf poultice applied 2-4 times daily over the injury site is recommended. Comfrey will greatly speed the healing and repair of any damaged tissue. Comfrey is also known as "Bone-knit".

Fracture Diagnosis and Management

A fracture is the medical term for a broken bone. It is not true that "if you can move the part (the joint or limb), then it is not broken. Pain will prevent some movement, but does not determine the difference between a fracture and a contusion. A fracture can be "simple" meaning that the bone has a single crack or "compound" with many cracks and pieces. There is no way to determine the exact nature of a fracture without the aid of an x-ray. A deformity in the shape or contour of the limb indicates a fracture or contusion with soft tissue bleeding if located along the middle or shaft of a long bone. A possible dislocation or severe sprain with or without a fracture if located at a joint. The hallmark of a fracture is extreme point tenderness or pain to the touch over the site of the break. Swelling over the break site is further evidence of a fracture. Another way to determine the presence of a fracture is to apply gentle torsion (twisting) or compression to the bone in question. Either of these will cause pain at the site of the fracture. Some suggest that using a tuning fork on a bony prominence will cause a vibration along the bone eliciting pain at the fracture site. I have found this tuning fork method to be only mildly accurate.

Treatment: Each fracture has several critical aspects to consider in management; 1) Correct the loss of circulation or nerve damage due to deformity of the fracture; 2) Prevent infection if the skin is broken at or near the fracture site; 3) Prevent further soft tissue damage; and 4) Obtain a reasonable alignment of bone fragments so that adequate healing takes place.

The first aid approach to a fracture is to "splint them as they lie". Be sure and check the pulses distally from the injury. Splinting should not cause the pulse to diminish. This is appropriate if you are able to obtain professional medical attention. However, if the injury occurs in a remote area or medical attention is unavailable, you may need to straighten gross deformities of angulated fractures with gentle in-line traction.

Before straightening, check the pulses beyond the fracture site on both sides of the person and check for any abnormal sensations (this can be done by gently poking the person with something sharp and questioning the quality of the sensation). The technique for straightening is done with tractioning along the shaft of the long bone holding on to the joints above and below the fracture site. After correcting the angulation (bend in the arm) the circulation should improve. Arteries and veins are hollow tubes and when they are bent around a corner

or angle they stretch and narrow decreasing the flow of
blood. Once the bend is
eliminated, the tube
opens back up and the
blood will flow normally
again. It may be diffi-
cult to feel a good
pulse if the person
is going into shock.
Compare the in-
jured side to the un-
injured side (if you

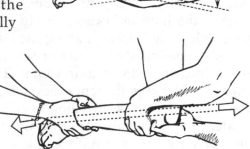

have that luxury). This will help you to better evaluate the
strength of the injured pulse.

Grossly angulated fractures can cause sharp ends of bone
to project against the skin surface. Even with careful padding, jostling along during an evacuation may cause one of
these bony spicules to penetrate the skin surface resulting in
an open fracture, increasing the chance of serious wound
and bone infection.

The chance of causing harm while straightening an angulated
fracture is extremely low. It is possible that a blood vessel or
nerve becomes trapped within the fracture site, but gentle re-
positioning into slight deformity should correct this. Monitor
the pulse for correction.

When splinting use padding to prevent skin damage. Pneu-
matic splints (inflatable) are available. In general, fractures are
splinted to immobilize the joint above and below the fracture
site. I recommending taking a first aid course to better learn
first aid basics. When a limb is properly splinted, the pain of
the fracture will decrease. If you are in doubt whether or not
there is actually a fracture, splint and treat for pain. Have
an x-ray taken. Avoid the use of the involved part for a
couple of days. If the pain has diminished then there was
likely no fracture. If there is still significant pain, then a fracture is more likely.

Treatment: Splint or cast as may be appropriate. I prefer a
splint that is removable so you can apply daily
CTR(Complete Tissue Repair) ointment, and comfrey tea
compresses. Comfrey (which is a main ingredient in CTR) is

known as a cell proliferate (increases cellular growth and repair). Take CTR syrup 3 times daily. Drinking carrot juice daily (3-6 cups) will speed healing. SuperNutrition taken 2-3 times daily (see page 217).

Open Fracture Management

Even a puncture wound or laceration near a broken bone is a cause for alarm. A wound near a fracture site can allow bacteria to enter the bone resulting in a serious bone infection. This type of wound requires aggressive cleansing as indicated on page 199 (see wound cleansing). The wound should not be closed as this increases the chance of infection. Wet dressings are best over an open wound. Soak the sterile dressing in an herbal infusion of Goldenseal and comfrey and cover the wound. Change this dressing twice daily.

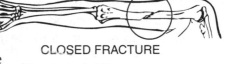

CLOSED FRACTURE

OPEN FRACTURE

Treatment: If a piece of bone is protruding from the skin, the break is called an "open fracture".

The first aid approach is to asses the distal pulse and splint the fracture in the position you find it and cover the wound with a sterile dressing, then seek medical attention. If you are unable to get medical assistance you will need to treat this injury yourself. Begin with cleaning the wound with aggressive irrigation and scrubbing with mild soap as described on page 199.

The aggressiveness of this cleansing should be done in such a manner that no further damage is caused, but the area must be cleansed and free of any dirt or germs. Use only enough pressure to control any bleeding and always use sterile gauze. Straighten any gross angulation of the fracture with gentle in-line traction. This will cause the protruding bone to disappear under the surface of the skin, unless the fragment is loose from the main bone. Remember you must clean this wound thoroughly before you set the bone.

Use Immune enhancing herbs to strengthen the body to fight infection. Herbal antiseptic tincture should be used over the wound. This will be painful but necessary to kill germs or bacteria. Do not cast or cover this type of wound, as you must watch and monitor the healing making sure there is no infection.

Diagnosis & Care protocols

Diagnosing injuries can be difficult without the aid of x-rays and if you lack experience. In evaluating the person, always compare the injured side to the non-injured side. Take the clothing off the injured side as well as the normal side and compare them. Look for swelling or a different shape. Use a light touch. Fractures and sprains are very tender and will not require rough palpation. A fracture will always cause swelling (the result of localized bleeding due to the trauma. Several days after an injury a bruise may appear on the surface or below the area (gravity helps it settle down hill). Do not be concerned about the spreading of a bruise. As the blood is displaced and spreads, the body is better able to reabsorb and clean it up.

BROKEN NECK OR BACK

If the victim cannot move his fingers readily, or if there is tingling or numbness in his hands, arms or shoulders, there is the possibility his neck has been broken.

If he can move his fingers but not his feet or toes, or if he has tingling or numbness in his legs, or pain in his back or neck, his back may be broken. Call for emergency medical assistance at once.

Do not let the victim attempt to move. The spinal cord extends through the neck and back vertebrae, and any movement may cause paralysis.

If the victim is not breathing, administer artificial respiration (see page 18), taking care to avoid all movement of the neck. If, to avoid further injury, the victim must be moved, carefully support his head and neck and move him lengthwise - not sideways (see illustration page 37 "moving victims).

Once the fracture and injuries have been stabilized assist the healing process through the use of herbal therapy.

Apply CTR ointment over affected area as you are able. More importantly, take CTR Syrup 3-5 times daily.

Drinking comfrey leaf or root tea - 3 to 6 cups per day is

advisable. A comfrey leaf poultice applied 2-4 times daily over the injury site is recommended.

If there has been damage to the spinal cord or peripheral nerves administer Nerve Repair Formula - 3-5 dropperfuls each day for 3 to 6 months.

NECK INJURY

Definition/Diagnosis: Neck injuries can be life threatening. The brain stem can extend down to the second and third cervical vertebrae. In fact a "hangman's fracture" of the 3rd cervical vertebra actually ruptures into the portion of the brain stem that controls breathing. The hanged-man suffocates for neurologic reasons rather than simply being choked. It is essential to protect the spinal cord from injury while examining the neck.

Treatment: Without moving the neck, gently palpate along the spinous processes (the bones you can feel from the back of the neck). If there is no tenderness, there is generally not any significant bone damage. If the person is unconscious, treat as if the neck is fractured. Splint the neck so that it is immobilized. If the neck is at an odd angle, it should be straightened with gentle traction-in-line, by pulling steadily and slowly on the head along the line in which you find the neck. Then move the neck to a neutral position in line with the spine. It is important that the neck is immobilized to prevent any broken bone fragments from cutting in to and damaging the spinal cord or nerve roots. Do not allow the person to move or be lifted until the neck is completely immobilized. The best technique for initial immobilization of the neck is gentle but firm holding of the persons head. A neck brace made of a towel or a rolled cloth can be used.

Fractures of the neck can be very unstable and must be evaluated by x-ray and stabilized for proper healing to occur.

Herbally: Use comfrey fomentations, drink comfrey tea (3-6 cups daily), or use CTR ointment and syrup that you'e made. Good dietary practices will definitely speed healing and recovery. Drinking plenty of carrot juice will decrease recovery time.

If you do not find any point tenderness on the spinal bones, but more of a generalized pain and spasming of the neck muscles, a moderate or severe sprain of the neck is likely.

You may want to make a neck brace as above. Lobelia can be used as a muscle relaxant and herbs for pain are beneficial. Follow the instructions for healing soft tissue injuries on page 260.

SPINAL INJURY

Definition/Diagnosis: Always check the entire spine when there has been a hard fall or traumatic impact or injury. For a quick neurologic check ask the person if there is any numbness or tingling anywhere. Check their grip strength on both sides and have them wiggle their toes and flex their feet up and down. Check the entire spine for point tenderness on the spinous processes (bony bumps down the center of the back). If you find something on the exam (pain, weakness, numbness, etc.), or even if the trauma seems severe, both the back and neck should be immobilized. Maintain firm hand control of the neck until the patient is placed on a rigid stretcher and evacuate the person to medical help. Of course, if you have the luxury of calling for professional medical help, always do that first. Immobilizing even a healthy person on a stretcher will cause back pain after 30 minutes. If you are in a remote area reassess the spine to ensure that immobilization is really necessary. You will have to use your common sense. If the person is not able to move an extremity or has lost sensation without an orthopedic injury to that limb, you must be very suspicious of a spinal cord injury. If these signs are not present then you are most likely dealing with muscle problems rather than a broken or disrupted spine. "The spine may be cleared" - this is a term which means that you may take them off of the rigid support.

Treatment: Treat herbally as indicated under "neck injury".

BACK PAIN

Definition/Diagnosis: Back pain effects 80% of adults at some time in their lives. Most cases of back pain are a result of simple muscle strain. If back pain persists for more than 72 hours or if the pain radiates into the legs, or if other symptoms such as unexplained weight loss occur consult with a healthcare practitioner that specializes in the treatment of back pain. If the person's pain is unrelenting and he has begun to or has lost bowel and bladder control this could be the result of a herniated disc and may require surgical repair. A healthy spine that is both strong and flexible will usually be self correcting. Often back pain can result from constipation (see page 51). In women, lower back pain can occur during menses or be the result of uterine or ovary problems. If the pain follows an injury and is accompanied by sudden loss of bladder or bowel control, if you have difficulty moving any limb, or if you feel numbness, pain, or tingling in a limb, do not move, but call for medical help immediately. You may have hurt your spinal cord.

Treatment: To relieve back and/or neck pain use alternating hot/cold hydrotherapy and massage in Deep Heat ointment (see "Healing Soft Tissue Injuries" see page 260). Spinal manipulation should only be performed by someone trained in the proper methods and precautions of spinal care. Gentle yoga stretches for the lower back are most beneficial. Herbal Pain Formula is useful. Valerian and Nerve Calm Formula (see page 232) and good herbal relaxants.

NECK PAIN

Definition/Diagnosis: There are many causes of neck pain. If the onset is traumatic in origin treat as you would in this section under sprains or strains or neck injury. If there is no traumatic origin and neck pain is accompanied with a headache and fever, refer to meningitis, page 171. If the person simply woke up with a kink or crick in their neck, consult with a chiropractor, massage therapist, or use the Twin Tennis Balls in Tandem therapy on page 263. Always look to and treat the cause.

COLLAR BONE (Clavicle)

Definition/Diagnosis: Evaluate for pain by palpating along the collarbone (clavicle). With trauma the clavicle can separate at either end, at the sternum (breastbone) or at the shoulder. Fractures are commonly at the mid-portion of the bone.

Treatment: Separations and fractures alike can be stabilized with a sling and swath. Always assess the distal pulses before and after putting on a sling or wrapping an injury. If because of your splint the pulse diminishes, you must readjust the splinting to insure good circulation. To make a sling, wrap material behind the neck then around the injured arm. Next take a wide cloth and wrap it around the outside of the injured arm across the body and under the uninjured side. This is designed to hold the arm next to the body, and is called a swath.

If the clavicle is fractured in the mid-portion, proper reduction of the fracture can be obtained using a figure-eight splint. Wrap the cloth around both shoulder crossing in a figure-eight behind the back. This should hold the shoulders back like a person standing "at attention". Using a sling will add stabilization and help with pain control. A swath will even further stabilize and thus reduce pain.

If the fracture is at the end of the clavicle near the shoulder, it may be hard to hold in its proper position. Treat with a sling and swath. In any clavicle fracture a sling will greatly help to reduce the pain. Keep the arm/clavicle in the sling and immobilized for two weeks. Keep the figure-eight splint on for 3 to 4 weeks. Do not, DO NOT allow the person to stoop the shoulders forward, this will allow the fractured ends to override each other. You really don't want an extra joint in the middle of the clavicle.

Herbally: Treat as you would any soft tissue injury. Use comfrey tea or CTR Syrup (see page 224) to speed the healing and reduce the inflammation. CTR Ointment or Deep Heat (see page 52) for muscle spasm. Use herbal pain formula (see page 233) as needed.

DISLOCATED JOINTS - general instructions

Do not attempt to move or set a dislocated joint unless you have been trained to do so. Get medical attention promptly. If you must move the victim, first use splints to immobilize the joint in the position in which you find it. If the person has a hip dislocation, call an ambulance or move him on a stretcher to a hospital emergency room. To reduce swelling and relieve pain, apply an insulated ice bag to the injured part. Use herbal pain formula as needed. Once the dislocation has been reduced, treat as you would a sprain with R.I.C.E., CTR ointment and syrup, etc.

SHOULDER

Definition/Diagnosis: Shoulder separations are classified as Grade I, II, and III depending on the severity. Grade I has tenderness over the acromio-clavicular joint (where the clavicle meets the top of the shoulder in the front). In a Grade I, ligaments are strained with no disruption or tearing. Grade II is a rupture of the two acromio-clavicular ligaments, which will result in a slight elevation of the clavicle. This elevation may be slight. There will be increased pain over the AC joint (acromio-clavicular joint) with weight bearing (lifting or pushing). A grade III strain is the disruption of both AC ligaments as well as the coraco-clavicular ligament. There is no strong evidence that Grade III separations do better with surgical repair than those without. Without surgery, you're left with a slight deformity at the end of the clavicle. Treat with the arm in a sling for 3 to 6 weeks. Mobilize the shoulder as soon as possible moving the shoulder in a figure-eight motion starting out with small circles (figure-eights) gradually increasing the range of motion to a full range of motion. Treat herbally with comfrey and CTR (see page 224) and herbs for pain as needed.

Shoulder dislocations are separations or displacements of the humerus from the shoulder socket moving either anterior or posterior and down. Anterior is by far the most common. Fractures of the head, or top part of the humerus may occur with a dislocation. A dislocation should be reduced as soon a possible. Muscle spasm and pain will continue to increase the longer the dislocation is allowed to remain untreated. Anterior dislocations may be identified by comparing the shoulder to the opposite side. The normal smooth rounded contour of the shoulder, which is on the outside is diminished or lost. With an anterior dislocation the lateral (outside) contour is sharply rectangular and the front (anterior) contour is very prominent. The arm will be held away from the body and any attempt at moving the arm will be very painful.

A numb area located just beneath the deltoid (shoulder) muscle means that the axillary nerve has been damaged. Numbness or tingling of the little finger could mean that the ulnar nerve has been damaged. Decreased sensation to the thumb, index, and middle finger may mean that the median nerve is injured. If you find any of these, there is an increased urgency to reduce the dislocation.

The best method of reducing the anterior dislocation of the shoulder is the Stimson Maneuver. There should be minimal pain using this technique. It usually takes at least 20 minutes for this method to work. There will be a sudden clunk as the shoulder goes back into the socket. There will be instant pain relief and the patient will be able to use the arm again (minimally). To perform this maneuver have the patient lie face down on a table so that the affect arm can hang over the edge. Using a wide cloth, wrap the forearm several times. Attach this wrap to a bucket or bag filled with 10-15 pounds of rocks or sand. Then allow gravity to gradually stretch the muscles until the shoulder relocates itself into the socket.

After the dislocation is reduced, place the arm in a sling and a swath wrapped around the arm and chest to hold the arm against the body for 3 weeks. If the person begins using the arm too soon, the shoulder will remain weak and unstable. In a young person, a sling and swath should be worn for 4 weeks before range of motion exercises begin. Keeping the arm in the sling longer than 4 weeks has no advantages.

Treat herbally as indicated on page 68 (beginning of ortho section).

SHOULDER BLADE (Scapula)

Definition/Diagnosis: Fractures of the scapula are generally due to a major trauma. Often multiple rib fractures, punctured lung(pneumothorax) or a heart contusion may accompany scapula fractures. Without an x-ray diagnosis is difficult. Be suspicious if there is point tenderness over the scapula, especially if it is there several days after the accident. A triangular swelling outlining the scapula indicates a fracture. This swelling is call Comolli's sign.

Treatment: Stabilize the arm and shoulder with a sling. Begin mobilizing the shoulder as soon as you can always working within the limits of pain. Treat herbally as indicated with other orthopedic injuries (see page 68).

UPPER ARM (Humerus)

Definition/Diagnosis: A fracture to the upper arm is associated with swelling and eventual bruising of the shoulder and upper arm. Displacement and severe angulation may require surgical repair. Severe pain will prevent normal movements of the shoulder. Humerus fractures heal themselves quite readily but can take 2 to 4 months to heal completely. Humeral shaft fractures at a point one third of the way up from the elbow may cause damage to the radial nerve, resulting in numbness to the forearm, thumb and index finger. This numbness generally lasts from 3 to 6 months and usually resolves on its own.

Treatment: If medical help and an x-ray machine are unavailable treat conservatively with a sling and a swath (see explanation under clavicle section, page 80). Always asses the distal pulses before and after putting on a sling or wrapping an injury. If because of your splint the pulse diminishes, you must readjust the splinting to insure good circulation. It is important that older people (55+, not to offend you) begin moving and mobilizing the shoulder as soon as possible to prevent adhesion (scar tissue) formation within the muscles resulting in a "frozen shoulder". Keep the arm in the sling from a few days to 6 weeks depending on how much displacement there was initially. If the person is over 30 begin mobilizing after two weeks. Younger people can be left in a sling for 4 weeks. Physical therapy should consist of range of motion movements such as circular elephant trunk motions and figure-eight motions while bending over. Raise the arm in front, to the side, and toward the rear. Move the shoulder "as if the person was wiping their bottom". All of these motions should be done by the person without someone forcing their arm through these motions.

Treat herbally: is indicated at the beginning of the orthopedic section, page 68.

ELBOW

Definition/Diagnosis: Fractures of the humerus just above the elbow and of the elbow itself (the olecranon process) can be very dangerous as bone fragments can seriously injure the nerves, blood vessels or articular surfaces of the bones in this area. The swelling involved in a fracture or dislocation can cause compression and more damage to the nerves than a sharp bone. Dislocations are more frequent in young adults and are of the result of extreme hyperextention. The appearance of a dislocation should be obvious when compared to the other side. This dislocation results in forcing the ulna backwards so that the olecranon process (the tip of the elbow) becomes very prominent.

Treatment: Reduction of a dislocation or setting of a fracture elbow should be done by an orthopedic specialist. If medical help is unavailable, the Stimson technique of reducing a hyperextension dislocation can be performed. Use herbs for pain and to relax the muscles before attempting to reduce the elbow. Lobelia taken orally (10 drops) and lightly rubbed into the painful elbow and surrounding muscles if effective. Lie the person face down (prone) with their arm bent at an angle over the edge of the table. Traction the wrist downward while gently pushing the olecranon to reduce the dislocation.

For both fracture and dislocation the arm should be set in a sling and held at a 120° angle. Because of the swelling setting the arm at 90° could cause nerve compression. Pad the elbow posteriorly (in the back) but not in the front. Feel the pulses in the wrists, if the pulse is decreased lower the arm down to where you get the strongest pulse. Splint for 3 weeks for a dislocation, then begin motion exercises. Follow instructions for Healing Soft Tissue Injuries as described on page 260, in addition to the herbal instructions at the beginning of the orthopedic section, page 68.

FOREARM (Radius/Ulna)

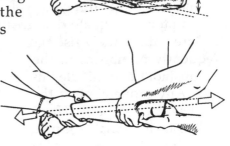

Definition/Diagnosis: Forearm fractures in children can generally be treated by reducing under x-ray (x-ray, set the bone, re-x-ray to see if it's right, etc.) and cast. Adults may require surgical repair. If neither option is available, set the bones if there is any displacement, by traction as diagrammed then splint.

Most fractures of the forearm are not complete and unstable. They will heal readily with only protective splinting. It is important that the arm is protected while it heals, as the bone is weakened during the healing process.

Treatment: Always assess the distal pulses before and after putting on a sling or wrapping an injury. If because of your splint the pulse diminishes, you must readjust the splinting to insure good circulation. Pad the splint well and keep splinted for 6 weeks immobilizing the elbow and the wrist. Ice and use the herbal recommendations as indicated on page 68.

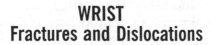

WRIST
Fractures and Dislocations

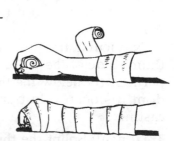

Definition/Diagnosis: Wrist fractures and dislocations are common in young adults when they fall with the arm and hand extended. The three most common problems are fractures of the navicular (also called scaphoid) bone, dislocation of the lunate, and perilunate dislocation. Navicular fractures often do not heal even with appropriate casting. This is in large part because when this bone fractures, its circulation is broken as well. Dislocations of the lunate or of the remaining carpals (the bones of the wrist) from the lunate would ideally be reduced, but without x-ray, expertise, and local anesthesia it is difficult.

Symptoms of lunate dislocation are pain in the wrist and frequently numbness in the thumb, index and middle fingers. Any movement of the wrist will elicit pain. There will be an abnormal bump on the palm side of the wrist at the crease, when compared to the other wrist. The numbness is due to pressure on the median nerve from the dislocated lunate bone. Reduce this dislocation by hold the wrist into extreme dorsiflexion (wrist flexed back - fingers toward elbow), traction while pushing the bone back into position. There is usually an obvious pop when it goes back into place.

Perilunate dislocations will have similar signs and symptoms however the knob will not be present. Rather there will be a slight deformity on the back side of the wrist. The technique of reduction is similar, with traction being applied to the wrist, while placing your thumb on the lunate bone pushing down while flexing the wrist. You should hear the bone snap back into place. The numbness should wear of within the next hour or so if the pressure is taken off the median nerve.

Navicular fractures will have pain particularly on the thumb side of the wrist. The entire wrist will be painful, but particularly below the thumb at the wrist. This fracture seldom dislocates, but is prone to not healing, even after casting.

Treatment: Splint the thumb and wrist, whether or not you were successful at reducing the dislocation. You may use an ace bandage or Unna paste dressing wrapped as illustrated. This is called a thumb spica wrap.

Use herbal and water therapies as detailed on page 68 at the beginning of the orthopedic section.

THUMB
Sprains and Fractures

Definition/Diagnosis: Injuries causing severe pain and swelling could be either a sprain or fracture. A severe sprain will cause loss of strength of the thumb for many weeks, even months. Swelling can be substantial with either injury. The first aid management is splinting until treatment by a physician can be arranged. In an extended survival situation, reduce any obvious deformity and hold in position with a thumb spica wrap. (See illustration above). Severe sprains and fractures can take 8 weeks to heal. Of course using herbs and water therapy will greatly reduce the healing time. For you natural healthcare zealots, just because you are using herbs and things are healing fast, don't get cocky and push the joint or injury too hard prematurely. It is always better to exercise caution and restraint rather than showing off how quickly you have healed.

HAND - Metacarpals and Fingers

Definition/Diagnosis: Fracture of the 1st metacarpal should be treated with a thumb spica wrap which will immobilize the entire wrist. The 5th metacarpal is the most common broken bone in the hand (called a boxer's fracture). A perfect reduction is not necessary, in fact up to 30 degrees of angulation is quite functional. If angulation of a fracture is very noticeable or extreme (x-ray of course is the only real way to tell), then the bones may need to be snapped back into place. Wrap and splint the hand for up to six weeks and treat as you would herbally with CTR, Comfrey and hot and cold hydrotherapy.

FINGERS - Fractures and Sprains

Definition/Diagnosis: Gross deviations of fingers should be corrected and the finger splinted in the neutral position (relaxed slightly bent). These deviations can be corrected by tugging and thus resetting the fracture or by placing a pencil or similar object between the fingers and using leverage to snap a deviated finger shaft back into place. A deviation at a joint is a dislocation and can easily be reduced by tugging on the finger. Swelling that is associated with "jammed" fingers can become permanent if you begin using the finger before adequate healing has taken place. After the acute injury, splint in a position with the finger slightly curved (the position of function) for at least three weeks. Then buddy splint to the adjacent finger for another two weeks.

A mallet finger deformity occurs when the distal extensor tendon is ruptured resulting in the end of the finger being held in a flexed position even though the rest of the finger is held straight. This type of injury can occur by an object hitting the tip of the finger or catching the finger in something like getting it snagged on a sheet while making a bed. The finger must be splinted so that the distal joint is immobile. The splint must be worn continuously for 6 to 8 weeks otherwise this tendon will not heal properly and the joint will remain in the flexed position. Do not let the finger drop back into flexion. After the eight weeks wearing a splint during activities that may offer a risk to re-injury is advised.

Finger injuries can be treated herbally just as other orthopedic injuries.

HIP - Dislocation and Fracture

Definition/Diagnosis: Hip injuries can be very serious because of the internal bleeding that can occur. Fractures of the hip cause pain in the anterior medial aspect (front and to the inside) of the thigh. In younger people dislocations may be associated with fractures, in older people fractures are very common and should be considered with any deformity or misplacement of the hip. If internal bleeding is suspected, cayenne tincture (1-2 dropperfuls) or cayenne powder mixed in water (1/2 to 1 tsp.) should be given. Cayenne is natures best tool to control bleeding whether internally or externally.

There are three main types of dislocations/ fractures to the hip. Posterior dislocations, anterior hip dislocations and central fracture/dislocations (where the head of the femur is driven through the hip socket into the pelvis. Posterior dislocations of are more common in healthy young adults. Posterior dislocations can cause injury to the sciatic nerve resulting in shooting pain and/or numbness down the back or side of the leg. This type of dislocation should be reduced within

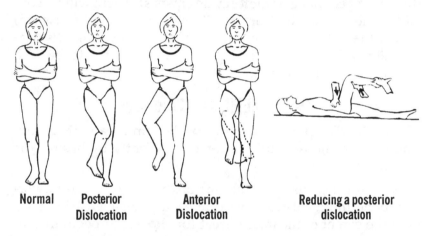

| Normal | Posterior Dislocation | Anterior Dislocation | Reducing a posterior dislocation |

24 hours. Continued pressure on the sciatic nerve can result in atrophy (wasting of the muscle) and loss of sensation to nearly the whole leg.

Treatment: To reduce a posterior dislocation, place the person on their back with the knee and hip in a 90° position. The line of the femur should point straight upwards. The thigh should be pulled steadily upwards while simultaneously rotating the femur externally.

A central fracture/ dislocation should be x-rayed to determine

Traction on the hip then rotate the hip externally (the foot will rotate along the midline of the body) causing the hip to relocate within the socket.

the extent of the damage and surgical repair and replacement of the fragments may be necessary. If medical care is not available, this type of injury can do a good job healing on its own resulting in a stable relatively painless joint. Apply light traction to the leg for comfort. After three weeks, begin moving about with the aid of crutches gradually increasing the weight put on the leg. Range of motion exercises are important from the beginning. This will help to mold the healing fragments into a smooth joint surface. Herbal therapies as described on page 68 are vitally important with this type of injury.

Anterior hip dislocations usually result from very forceful accidents (plane or motorcycle crashes). There will be considerable lateral rotation (the foot will be tilted outward) when the patient is lying on his back. Reduce this dislocation similarly to a posterior hip dislocation but rotate the limb inward instead of outward.

THIGH (FEMUR) - Fractures

Definition/Diagnosis: Fractures of the femur can occur from the knee to the hip and are rated differently by orthopedic specialists.

Treatment: Because the muscles of the thigh are so powerful, bone fragments can override each other increasing pain and the extent of the injury. Treat for shock and begin to gently traction the leg in-line. You can be creative using a trucker's hitch to keep the leg traction. Tractioning will establish normal length and configuration of the muscles allowing the membranes to tighten. This will decrease the bleeding which occurs with this injury. Tractioning is also the best way to reduce the pain. After several days you may buddy splint the leg to the other leg. Prolonged pressure from cord cloth can lead to necrosis (death) of the skin of the ankle due to the pressure. Treat herbally with comfrey tea, CTR, gentle massage, direction of energy etc. (see page 68).

PATELLA (knee cap)

Definition/Diagnosis: The knee cap usually dislocates laterally (to the outside). This dislocation results in a locking of the knee and the knee cap bumped off to the side makes this diagnosis obvious.

Treatment: Relocate the patella by flexing the hip and the knee, then straighten the knee and the patella usually snaps back into place by itself. If it doesn't, just push the knee cap into place while straightening the knee on the next try. The knee should be splinted with the knee slightly flexed. The patient should be able to walk without any threat of re-injury, re-dislocation or problems.

KNEE - Sprain, Dislocations, Fracture

Definition/Diagnosis: The initial care of an acute sprain is described on page 70 under Joint Injury- Acute Onset. If the pain in the knee is severe, then you could be looking at a tear to the ligaments, tendons, cartilage, and/or synovial membranes. There could also be fractures or dislocations involved. Intensity of pain is of course very subjective. Significant deformity means that a dislocation may have occurred and disruption of the nerve and blood flow could be impeded. Check the pulses on the top of the foot to assess blood flow. Also check the sensation of the feet for nerve sensation. If the pulses are OK, splint the knee as it lies. If the pulse is weaker on the injured side, get a helper to hold the knee while you grip the ankle with one hand and the calf with the other. Traction in-line while you gently flex the knee to see if you can reposition it better. If the pain is too intense, you meet resistance, or you just can't do it, splint the knee as best you can to make the person comfortable and transport for medical help as soon as you can. Even without obvious deformity, an immediate or continuous complaining about significant pain means that you should have the person evaluated medically. If on the other hand, in two hours, the next morning or in two days, the person feels better and wants to walk, let him. Walk using a cane on the side of the good leg.

Treatment: RICE the knee - Rest, Ice, Compress and Elevate. Treat herbally for pain, inflammation and to speed tissue repair.

ANKLE - Sprains, Dislocations, Fractures

Definition/Diagnosis: Fractures of the ankle on either side is associated with a dislocation. Splint the ankle to stabilize. A flail ankle, caused by complete disruption of the ankle ligaments, easily slops back into position and can be held in place with a trough-like splint. Allow the patient to rest after the injury before trying to walk. Let pain be you gauge as to how much pressure to put on the ankle. A severe sprain and a fracture can be equally painful.

Use a SAM Splint as an ankle wrap.

Treatment: RICE (Rest, Ice, Compress, Elevate) the ankle. Keep the ankle wrapped in an ace bandage, or ankle brace. Use hot & cold hydrotherapy and treat herbally for pain and tissue repair. Begin using a cane when able.

You can also use a belt, ace bandage or a cloth.

FOOT/TOES

Definition/Diagnosis: Stubbed toes (ooouch!) can be buddy splinted to provide pain relief. If they have been stubbed to the extent that they deviate off to the side at a crazy angle, reposition it before you buddy splint (tape). To reposition, you can use a pencil (or similar object) on the opposite side of the toe using it as a fulcrum to snap the toe back into alignment (sounds brutal doesn't it). Place some cotton or gauze material between toes to prevent rubbing. Then tape the fractured toe to the adjacent toe.

Severe pain in the arch of the foot or in the metatarsals can be caused by either a fracture or sprain. RICE as described above. Minor injuries will decrease in pain within a short time (a couple of days) while fractures may take weeks to decrease in pain. Treat herbally for pain, inflammation and tissue repair.

Chapter 5

CHEST & RESPIRATORY PROBLEMS

ALLERGIES

Allergies result when the body responds inappropriately to a normal substance. Almost anything can cause allergies, from mold, pollens, dust, chemicals, foods, etc. Often environmental allergies can be controlled by eliminating the most common food allergens, milk/dairy, eggs, peanuts, wheat, soy, cashews, shellfish, strawberries, beef, pork, corn, and chocolate. Because of modern hybrids, today's wheat is higher in gluten than ever before. Allergies, asthma, etc. often can be entirely eliminated by omitting all wheat and gluten products from the diet. Results are often seen within 2 to 3 days.

Anaphylactic Shock or Anaphylaxis is an allergic reaction that is so severe that it can kill within minutes. Insect bites or stings can cause this in some. More typically anaphylaxis results from a drug allergy. Treat with an injection of epinephrine delivered through an "Epi-Pen" Epinephrine Auto Injector. This should be kept on hand if you are known to have severe allergic reactions to bites or stings. And of course, stay away from drugs unless you are under medical supervision that is able to deal with such emergencies.

Treatment: Lobelia tincture should be used at the first sign of an allergic reaction (1 to 10 dropperfuls, begin with one dropperful then give more every 30 seconds as needed). Too much lobelia can cause vomiting, but that is really nothing to be concerned over as this will empty the stomach. Lobelia is in no way harmful to the body. Double or triple the intake of SuperNutrition. Take three times daily Anti-Plague Formula or Immune Boost. Take Allergy Formula 3-4 capsules every four hours as needed to reduce symptoms. Digestive enzymes are often very helpful and bee pollen has helped many. Reduce stress in your life. Food and/or environmental allergies can require some detective work or visiting someone trained in BioSET Allergy Elimination or muscle testing techniques for identifying and eliminating allergies.

ASTHMA

Definition/Diagnosis: Asthma is a lung disease that causes obstruction of the airways. During an asthma attack, spasms in the muscles surrounding the bronchi impede the outward and inward movement of air. There are two types of asthma prevalent today, spasmodic and inflammatory. Spasmodic asthma is the type of asthma that was most common 40 years ago. It results is spasms of the respiratory muscles causing airway distress. Inflammatory asthma on the other hand is a result of pollution and toxicity being breathed in, resulting in the airways to be irritated. It is kind of like having hives in the airways. Any additional irritation can cause swelling and close up the bronchial tubes.

Treatment: 1) Spasmodic Asthma - use Lung formula (lobelia, peppermint, ephedra), and 2) Inflammatory Asthma - immune boost, anti-plague formula, Pau d'arco, and dietary. Inflammatory Asthma is now more common and does not respond well to bronchial dilator herbs. Anyone serious about helping asthma must stop **all** dairy consumption. Good dietary practices are essential for the long term management of asthma (see page 243). One dropperful of lobelia tincture is very helpful during an acute asthma attack. Mullein oil is a powerful remedy for bronchial congestion. This oil will stop coughs, unclog bronchial tubes and helps clear up asthma attacks. Mullein and Lobelia oil as made by Western Botanicals is very effective. Comfrey tea 2 to 3 times daily is useful in healing the lungs.

For acute respiratory distress, massage lobelia tincture between the shoulder blades, across the rib cage, and throughout the chest and ribs.

Lobelia Purge for Asthma: This procedure can be used to help chronic asthma. It may seem dramatic but it really is quite effective. Drink 1 cup of peppermint tea, after 10 minutes take 1 teaspoon lobelia tincture. Every 10 minutes take 1 teaspoon of lobelia tincture until vomiting begins. Vomiting may last several hours and will bring up all kinds of mucus. Often this alone will take care of serious chronic asthma.

BREATHING - RAPID (Hyperventilation or Tachypnea)

Definition/Diagnosis: Rapid breathing or hyperventilation can represent either a serious medication condition (such as diabetes) or can be the result of a harmless panic attack. High altitude stress can result in hyperventilation.

A feeling of panic which results in very rapid shallow breathing causes the victim to lose excessive amounts of carbon dioxide from the bloodstream. The resulting change in the acid-alkaline balance of the blood (respiratory alkalosis) will cause a numb feeling around the mouth, in the extremities, and if the breathing pattern persists, it can even lead to violent spasms of the hands and feet and loss of consciousness. This is a form of hysteria which appears in teenagers and healthy young adults.

Treatment: Have the person re-breath their own air from a paper bag or stuff sack (no plastic bags). Also give 6-30 drops of lobelia tincture. They need to be reassured and told to slow down the breathing. Often by explaining what will happen to them if they continue (i.e. they'll pass out), you can get them to slow down and relax. Be very calm as you deal with this person. It's fine for them to take long deep breaths. It is rapid breaths that cause the loss of so much carbon dioxide.

BRONCHITIS
see also pneumonia or asthma

Definition/Diagnosis: Bronchitis can be the acute or chronic inflammation of the mucous membranes of the bronchial tubes. It is generally caused by poor diet and poor bowel function (see constipation). Relieving the effects of bronchitis will not heal it. Bronchitis usually develops from a cold that settles into the lungs and if not corrected can lead to pneumonia or tuberculosis.

Treatment: Comfrey and almonds are specific for bronchitis. Use comfrey tea or CTR syrup (see page 224). Correct constipation herbally (see constipation, page 51). A lobelia purge as described under asthma will clear the mucus out of the chest (see page 95). Ginger and/or mullein fomentation over chest area is effective in loosening phlegm. Cayenne pepper is very effective for cutting the phlegm as are chickweed, comfrey, marshmallow root or mullein.

Lobelia tincture or Lung Formula 10 to 20 drops 2-3 times per day.

Bad attacks use 1 tsp. to 1 Tbs. lobelia or lung formula.

A hot vapor or steam bath followed by a cold shower or sponging is effective in the healing process.

COUGHING

Definition/Diagnosis: Coughing can range from a mild tickle in the throat to coughing up blood which would be indicative of pneumonia or bronchitis. Always look to what the underlying cause may be. Coughing in and of itself is just a symptom, but could be an important sign in diagnosis. A productive cough (producing mucus) that persists for months and tends to recur year after year is characteristic of chronic bronchitis. Smokers cough is obviously associated with persistent irritation.

Treatment: One or more of the following remedies can be very effective in treating this symptom.

1. Lobelia tincture or Lung Formula 10-15 drops 3 times daily or as needed.

2. Plantain tincture - 1-2 dropperfuls 3 times daily

3. Gargle with a tea made from Herbal Tooth Powder (see page 229).

4. Onion Cough Syrup (4-5 sliced onion cooked down with 1/2 cup honey, strain then add the juice of one lemon).

HICCUPS

Hiccups can be started by a variety of causes and are generally self-limited. Several approaches to relieve them may be used. Have the victim hold his breath for a long as possible or re-breath air from a paper bag or stuff sack (no plastic bags). This causes a rise in the carbon dioxide level and will help to stop the hiccup mechanism. Drinking 5 to 6 ounces of ice water fast sometimes works; one may also close his eyes and press firmly on the eyeballs to stimulate the vagal nerve to stop hiccups. Another method that my sons swear by is done by plugging your ears and nose then swallowing three times real hard. This is done by first putting a mouthful of water in your mouth and holding your nostrils shut with your thumbs and your ears with your index fingers. The herb lobelia in small qualities can calm a spasming diaphragm reflex. Use 3 to 10 drops of tincture directly in the mouth. Try also a spoon full of sugar.

HYPERVENTILATION

Definition/Diagnosis: Hyperventilation is a common complication of emotional upset and most often affects anxious, high strung persons who unknowingly breathe too rapidly. This disturbs the normal balance of carbon dioxide in the blood. The result is tingling and spasms of the fingers and toes and a peculiar numbness around the mouth. These symptoms make the victim still more anxious, and thus more hyperventilation results. The patient's color and pulse remain good.

Treatment: This is not a dangerous condition and can usually be helped by reassurance and this simple measure: have the person breathe slowly for ten minutes, occasionally longer, in a paper (not plastic) bag held tightly over his mouth and nose. Give the person a dose or dropperful of lobelia tincture or Bach Flower Rescue Remedy. Nerve Calm may also be used, but is not as fast acting as the others.

CHEST INJURIES

Definition/Diagnosis: Broken ribs can result after a blow to the chest, such as being hit with an object or trauma from an auto accident. Even a severe sneeze or cough can crack a rib. Broken ribs will be exquisitely tender at the site of the fracture with even the lightest touch. Deep breathing will aggravate the pain as will coughing, sneezing and of course laughing.

Wrapping the chest with a strap or band will provide some relief and prevent rib movement. However, it is very important that breathing and cough are easy. The cough reflex will keep the lungs clear and free from accumulation of fluid. Tying a large towel or T-shirt works pretty well. A fractured rib usually takes 6 to 8 weeks to heal. You know you're healed when you can enjoy a good laugh.

A similar pain can be caused from a tear of the intercostal muscles or a separation of the cartilage from the rib near the sternum or breast bone. Treat the same as a rib fracture. Each of these heal in generally 3 to 4 weeks.

Flail chest is the result of several adjacent ribs being broken in more than one location. This can cause a section of the chest wall to literally detach itself. It is held in place by the muscles and skin. This section of the chest wall can bulge out when the person exhales instead of contracting as the chest normally would. It can also move in when the rest of the chest expands during inhalation.

Broken ribs usually heal on their own inspite of the movement caused by breathing or a flail chest. The pain of a broken rib can be so intense that it feels as though the lung could be punctured at any minute. This is not likely to happen, but if it does, there is the chance that air will leak into the chest cavity causing a pneumothorax. This can lead to significant respiratory distress seen as cyanosis (a blue discoloration of the skin due to inadequate oxygen in the blood). Crepitation (a dry crackling sound and sensation) can form in the skin. This crackling sensation is very noticeable when running the fingers over the skin in the upper part of the chest. It is not painfull, but it indicates that a pneumothorax has occurred. A pneumothorax can resolve on its own or it can expand causing death. This situation can be a life and death emergency that is best handled by those trained to deal with this. Similarly, bleeding into the lung tissue can result in a hemothorax which can either resolve on its own or progress to death. Cyanosis and difficult breathing is also present in a hemothorax.

Treatment: Treat all of these conditions similarly with herbs for pain, CTR syrup and/or comfrey tea. Avoid unnecessary movement. Have the person hold their hand or a soft object against their chest when coughing to prevent rib movement and to help decrease the pain. Sitting will be the most comfortable position, even for sleeping. Use cayenne powder in water (1/2 to 1 tsp. in 1 cup of water) every 1/2 to 1 hour for both a pneumothorax and a hemothorax. A comfrey plaster or fomentation over the rib cage is appropriate.

OPEN (Sucking) CHEST WOUND

Definition/Diagnosis: If an object such as a bullet or knife enters the chest puncturing the rib cage and lung, a sucking chest wound can result. Air can pass in and out the hole with each breath. A victim with an open chest wound below the nipple line may also have an injury to the liver or spleen. Breathing will be painful and difficult. A sucking sound may be heard with each breath. Bubbles may be seen at the wound site. Crackling sounds may be heard or felt near the injury.

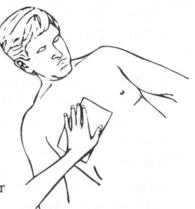

Treatment: Seal the opening immediately with any airtight substance (plastic works well, or gauze covered with Vaseline, CTR ointment or honey). Give the person 1 to 2 dropperfuls of cayenne tincture. Tape the gauze or plastic on three sides creating a flutter valve that will allow air to escape on exhalation. Call 911, get help. If an object is stuck in the chest, do not remove it. Apply several layers of dressings, clothing, etc. on the sides of the object to help stabilize it until help arrives.

PNEUMONIA - BRONCHITIS

Definition/Diagnosis: Infection of the airways in the lung (bronchitis) or infection in the air sacks of the lung (pneumonia) will cause very high fever, persistent coughing frequently producing phlegm stained with blood, and will cause extreme fatigue.

Treatment: Keep the person well hydrated, as fever and coughing lead to dehydration. Do not bundle the person with a high fever in blankets as this will drive the temperature only higher. The shivering cold feeling should not be trusted in gauging temperature. Use the back of your hand or a thermometer. Drinking an abundance of herbal teas such as peppermint & elder flower tea will keep the mucus from plugging up sections of the lungs.

Use the Cold Sheet Treatment, see page 248. Encourage the person to breath deeply several times each day. Force all the air out then inhale as deeply as possible. Repeat this 5 - 10 times or more.

Immune Boost Formula 1-2 dropperfuls 4-6 times daily

Anti-Plague Formula 1 tsp. To 1 Tbs. 4-6 times daily

Deep Heat rubbed into the chest or an old fashion mustard plaster can be effective in opening up the breathing

Plantain tincture 1-2 dropperfuls in hot water 4-5 times daily

Yarrow Tea 1 cup an hour until the fever breaks

Cayenne Tincture 5-6 drops 3 times daily

Garlic raw 5-8 cloves daily.

Do as much as you can and you will be pleased with your results.

PULMONARY CHILLING

Definition/Diagnosis: Sometimes called "frozen lung", occurs when breathing rapidly at very cold temperatures, generally below -20°F. There is burning pain, sometimes cough of blood, frequently asthmatic wheezing and with irritation of the diaphragm, pain in the shoulder and upper stomach that may last for two weeks.

Treatment: Treat with bedrest, steam inhalations of elecampane or pleurisy root tea, drinking 10-12 cups of water or herb tea daily, humidification of the living area and no smoking or being around those smoking. Avoid this condition by using parka hoods, face masks or breathing through mufflers which results in re-breathing warmed, humidified, expired air.

PULMONARY EMBOLUS

Definition/Diagnosis: A pulmonary embolus is a blood clot breaking loose from its point of origin, normally from a leg or pelvic vein, which then lodges in the lung after passing through the heart. When serious this condition results in shortness of breath, rapid breathing, with a dull pain under the breast bone. There may be a cough, bloody sputum, fever, and very sharp chest pain. This condition can be fatal if over 50% of the lung circulation is blocked.

Treatment: This usually resolves on its own within a couple of days. Drink teas that will support the lungs, such as pleurisy root, elecampane, and comfrey. Lobelia can maximize breathing. CTR syrup will aid and speed repair and recovery.

THROAT (Something Caught in it)

If something is caught in the throat (pharynx), it may obstruct swallowing or breathing or both. If only swallowing is obstructed, the person should proceed calmly as possible to the nearest hospital emergency room.

If the object obstructs the airway and breathing, treat for choking (see page 27).

Occasionally a person can experience the sensation of a lump in the throat that becomes chronic. This is often due to a lack of potassium. Use the Potassium Broth (Potato Peeling Broth) 3 to 6 cups daily as described on page 234. A fomentation of Mullein and Lobelia is also very helping in providing quick relief. (3:1 ratio).

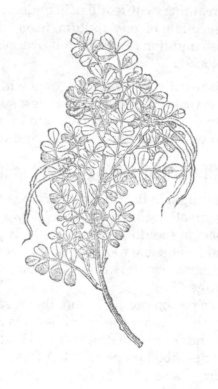

Chapter 6

EAR, EYE & NOSE PROBLEMS

EARACHE - in general

Definition/Diagnosis: Pain in the ear can come from many sources, including trauma, a foreign body, infection in the middle or outer ear, allergy, dental problems, TMJ dysfunction and swollen lymph nodes. This type of ear pain can be elicited by pushing on the knob at the front of the ear (the tragus) or pulling on the ear lobe. Tugging on the ear will not cause pain if the person has an middle ear infection. With a middle ear infection often there will be a history of head congestion and swollen or tender lymph nodes in the neck near the ear. If the skin above the swelling is red, the person probably has an infected skin abscess. The pain from an abscess is so localized, that confusion with an ear infection is rarely a problem. One or more tender lymph nodes can hurt to the extent that confusion of the exact source of pain may be in doubt. Swollen, tender nodes in the neck are usually associated with a sore throat, with severe Otitis externa or with infections of the skin in the scalp. Dental caries or cavities, can hurt like it is coming from the ear. Sometimes you can see these cavities with a pen light, otherwise tap each tooth to determine if it may be the source of pain.

OTITIS EXTERNA (Outer ear infection)

Definition/Diagnosis: This is commonly referred to as "swimmers ear". The external canal of the ear usually becomes inflamed from conditions of high humidity, accumulation of ear wax, or contact with contaminated water. Scratching the ear after picking your nose or scratching elsewhere can be a source of this common infection.

Treatment: Prevent cold air from blowing against the ear. Warm packs against the ear and putting in warm herbal ear oil. A very versatile ear oil can be made by soaking mullein leaf and garlic in extra virgin olive oil. Herbs for pain may be helpful. If a fever develops, the pain becomes severe, or the neck tissues or lymph nodes begin to swell begin using Immune Boost (page 230), Anti-Plague (page 219) or other immune supporting herbs. Drink plenty of water and/or herbal tea (Red raspberry or Yarrow). Use herbs for pain as necessary (Pain formula, white willow, valerian, passionflower). There is the old remedy of baking an onion that is cut in half until soft. Cool enough to allow you to put each half over each ear (or just one). Then wrap to hold the heat in. This is kind of messy but the warmth and the onion juice are very soothing and healing.

OTITIS MEDIA (common earache - middle ear)

Definition/Diagnosis: This condition will be present in a person who has sinus congestion and possible drainage from allergy or infection. The ear pain can be excruciating. Fever will often be intermittent, going up and down from normal to 103°F. Fever is a good indication that the infection may be bacterial. The eustachian tube leading from the oral cavity to the middle ear becomes clogged, usually with mucus, preventing drainage from the ear. Infants who sleep with a bottle of milk will often clog this tube up. The pain is associated with pressure against the ear drum. If the eardrum ruptures the pain will reduce immediately and the fever will drop. The hearing will be effected temporarily, however a ruptured ear drum heals rapidly.

Treatment: You may assist this healing with herbal ear oil or CTR oil (see page 224). If you were looking at the ear drum with an otoscope, it would be red and bulging from the pressure or sucked back by a vacuum in the middle ear.

Many people complain of hearing loss and think that they have wax or a foreign body in the ear, when in fact the middle ear is full of fluid. Besides the pain, the key to diagnosis is congestion in the head and fever. Protect the ear from cold and position the head so that the ear is directed upwards. Warm packs to the ear are helpful.

Garlic oil, Mullein oil, or Deep Heat oil 4-5 drops in the ear, then place a piece of clean cotton in the ear. Take Immune Boost hourly. 4-5 drops of Nerve Calm Formula in the ear will help with equilibrium problems, hearing loss or nerve damage. Massage the neck downward with Deep Heat ointment or Mullein/Lobelia oil. This will help to drain the lymph nodes.

EYE PATCH and BANDAGING TECHNIQUES

If evidence of infection is present, do not use an eye patch or splint, but have the person wear dark glasses, a wide brimmed hat, or take other measures to decrease light exposure. (See page 107, conjunctivitis)

Eye patch techniques must allow for gentle closure of the eyelid and should prevent any blinking activity. Sometimes both eyes must be patched for this to succeed, although this is usually a hardship for the person. Simple strips of tape holding the eyelids shut may suffice. In case of trauma, an annular ring of cloth may be constructed to pad the eye without pressure over the eyeball. A simple eye patch with oversize gauze or cloth may work fine, as the bone of the orbital rim (eye socket) around the eye acts to protect the eyeball which is recessed.

Serious injury requires patching both eyes, as movement in the uninjured eye will cause the injured eye to move. Have the person keep the head elevated slightly at rest after an eye injury. A severe blow to one eye may cause temporary blindness in both eyes which can resolve in hours to days. Obviously, a person with loss of vision should be treated by a physician if possible. Eye dressings must be removed, or at least changed, in 24 hours.

If the victim has suffered a corneal abrasion, or after removing a foreign body, the best splint is the tension patch. Start by placing two gauze pads over the shut eye, requesting the person to keep his eyes closed until the bandaging is complete. The person may help hold the gauze in place. Three pieces of one inch wide tape are ideal, long enough to extend from the center of the forehead to just below the cheek bone. Fasten the first piece of tape to the center of the forehead, extending the tape diagonally downward across the eye patch. The second and third strips are applied parallel to the first strip, one above and the other below. This dressing will result in firm splinting of the bandaged eye.

EYE ABRASION

Abrasions (or scrape) may be caused by a glancing blow from a wood chip, a swinging branch, or even blowing dirt, embers, ice or snow. The involved eye should be washed with an herbal eyewash (3-5 times daily). Make sure a foreign body has not been overlooked.

BLUNT TRAUMA TO THE EYE

Definition/Diagnosis: The immediate treatment is to immobilize the injured eye as soon as possible by patching both eyes and moving the person only by stretcher. Double vision could mean that there is a skull fracture near the eye or that there is a problem within the central nervous system. Double vision is sometimes caused by swelling behind the eyelid. A collection of blood in the anterior chamber of the eye called a hyphema may appear. The blood settles in front of the pupil, behind the cornea and has a distinct fluid level.

Treatment: Patch both eyes and take the person to a physician. Movement of one eye effects the other, so you really do need to patch both eyes. Transport the person with the head up from 45° to 90° to allow the blood to pool at the lower edge of the chamber. Check the eye twice daily for drainage which might indicate an infection. Treat herbal with Immune Boost (page 230) and/or Anti-Plague Formula (page 219) and/or Echinacea/Goldenseal combination (50/50). Use herbal pain formula (page 233). The person should avoid grimacing and thus squeezing the injured eye, which can compromised the eye even more. Apply herbal eyewash for pain of lacerations. Use CTR ointment and syrup to speed repair and healing. A comfrey poultice over the eye twice daily without any heat is appropriate. Dr. John Upledger in his book, *Your Inner Physician and You*, describes using a technique called V-spread in treating an eye injury. See Energy and Healing, page 263.

Severe injury to one eye can cause the other eye to become blind due to "sympathetic ophthalmia", which is probably an allergic response to eye pigment of the injured eye entering the victim's blood stream.

CONJUNCTIVITIS (Pink Eye)

Definition/Diagnosis: Conjunctivitis often is due to a blocked tear duct that prevents adequate drainage allowing an infection or inflammation of the eye surface. The eye will feel scratchy and will often feel like something is in the eye. The sclera (whites of the eye) will be red. Generally the eye will be matted shut in the morning with pus or granular matter. Infections are generally caused by bacteria, but viral infections also occur. Viral infections tend to have a blotchy red appearance over the sclera, while bacterial infections have a generalized red appearance. The drainage in bacterial infections tends to be pus, while viral infections tend to be watery. Allergic conjunctivitis results in a faint pink coloration and a clear drainage and is usually associated with other symptoms of allergy such as runny nose, no fever and no lymph node enlargement. With viral or bacterial look for fever and lymph node enlargement in the neck. Be sure that a foreign object is not the cause of the red eye.

Treatment: Wash the eye with herbal eyewash (eyebright, bayberry bark, Goldenseal and red raspberry leaf made into a tincture, see page 228). Wash every two hours dabbing to removed pus and excess secretions. This will unblock any clogged tear ducts. Herbal Eyewash Tincture - 4 to 10 drops in an eyecup of distilled or purified water, rinse eye/s hourly for conjunctivitis(pink eye) or 3 times daily for long term use. This will help sore, tired, infected eyes and poor vision. An old curative method that is still effective today is to simply chop onions and allow the juices to get into your eyes. You'll have a good cry and heal your eyes.

CONTACT LENSES

Definition/Diagnosis: As more and more people are wearing contact lenses there are several problems associated with them. There are two basic types of lenses. Hard or rigid lenses are usually smaller and does not extend beyond the iris, and soft lenses which extend beyond the iris into the whites of the eyes (the sclera). Hard lenses should not be left in the eye for more than 12 hours, as this may cause the cornea to ulcerate. While not serious, it is very painful but usually resolves within a day. If this condition associated with hard lenses does not resolve in 24 hours you may be looking at a corneal laceration, foreign body or eye infection. Check for a foreign body and if found treat appropriately.

If a laceration or infection is suspected treat with an herbal eyewash every 2 hours or at least 3-5 times daily. If herbal eyewash tincture is unavailable, a tea (infusion) made of eyebright and/or red raspberry is effective. Goldenseal is added to the eyewash for its antibiotic effect.

Eye pain may come from the migration or slipping of the lens into one of the recesses of the conjunctive, or they may simply notice the loss of vision correction in that eye. If someone exclaims "I've lost my contact!". Don't neglect looking in the eye for it. Examine the eye as described in the section on foreign bodies in the eye. If it is a hard lens and is loose, slide it over the pupil and allow the person to remove it as they usually do. If the lens adheres to the eye, rinse with an irrigation solution or clean water and try again. If a corneal abrasion exists or occurs, patch the eye as indicated after the lens is removed. A soft lens may generally be squeezed between the fingers and simply pops off.

Treatment: If the person is unconscious, the hard lenses will have to be removed. If a small suction cup for this purpose is not available there are two techniques which can be employed. The vertical technique is done by moving the lens to the center of the eye over the pupil. Then press down on the lower lid, over the lower edge of the contact lens. Next squeeze the eyelids together, thus popping the lens out between them. In the lateral technique, the lens is slid to the outside corner of the eye. By tugging on the skin of the face near the eye in a downward and outward(lateral) direction, the lens can pop over the skin edge and easily be removed. After the lenses are removed store in a safe place. Hard lenses should be wrapped securely so they won't rattle and be scratched. Soft lenses should be placed in saline solution to prevent dehydration (3/8 oz salt to 1/2 cup water). Use patients solution if available. Label contacts left and right. Use Herbal Eyewash 6-8 drops diluted in distilled water in an eyecup to rinse the eye every hour or until soreness abates.

FOREIGN BODY - Something's in My Eye

Treatment: The initial step in examining the painful eye is to remove the pain. Have the patient open the eye and look straight ahead. Very carefully shine a pen light at the cornea (outer globe of the eye). Go from one side to the next to see if a minute speck becomes visible. By moving the light back and forth, you may see movement of a shadow on the iris of the eye and thus confirm the presence of a foreign body.

To examine the eye, first check under the eyelids. Pull down the lower lid and turn back the upper lid. You may roll the eyelid up with a clean cotton swab and thus examine the eye as well as the eyelid. If the speck is on either lid, try to remove it by touching it lightly with the corner of a clean cloth or cotton swab. If the speck is on the eye itself, usually the normal tearing reaction will wash a speck out. If the speck or foreign body is on the surface of the eye, gently prod it with the cotton swab handle until it is loosened. The surface of the eye will indent under the pressure of the scraping action. The surface of the cornea will even be scratched in this maneuver, but it will heal quickly. Once the foreign body has been dislodged, if it does not stick to the wooden or plastic handle of the swab, but slips loose along the surface of the eye, use the cotton portion to touch it for removal. Foreign bodies stuck in the cornea can be very stubborn and resist removal. Leave stubborn foreign bodies for removal by a physician or someone trained in eye procedures. If you have a difficult time removing a foreign body from the surface of the cornea, place a bandage over both eyes and take the person to the doctor. It is important to cover both eyes. If only one eye is covered, the injured eye will move when the uninjured eye moves in looking about.

If the eye has been pierced by a foreign object, do not attempt to remove it, but seek immediate professional medical attention.

Once the eye has been treated or the speck removed, treat with Herbal Eyewash (see page 228). Rinse the eyes thoroughly 3-5 times daily.

GLAUCOMA

Definition/Diagnosis: Glaucoma is the rise of pressure within the eyeball (intraocular pressure increase). The most common form of glaucoma (open angle glaucoma) generally is not encountered until after the age of 40. The patient will note halos around lights, mild headaches, loss of vision to the sides (peripheral vision), and loss of the ability to see well at night. The external eye appears normal. Onset is usually gradual.

Treatment: Include warm compresses of eyebright tea and chamomile tea placed directly over the eye. Bilberry herb taken internally and herbal eye wash.

Acute glaucoma (narrow angle glaucoma) is much less common. It is characterized by a rapid rise in pressure of the fluid within the eyeball causing blurred vision, severe pain in the eye, even stomach pain. This situation can be a surgical emergency. Certain decongestant and medicines can cause or trigger acute glaucoma. READ the side effect of drugs before taking them.

SPONTANEOUS SUBCONJUNCTIVAL HEMORRHAGE

Definition/Diagnosis: This condition looks alarming but the person usually states that it doesn't hurt. There is bright bleeding over a portion of the white of the eye. It spreads out over a period of 12 - 48 hours, then reabsorbs slowly over the next 7 to 21 days, then turns yellowish as the blood is reabsorbed. Some state a vague feeling of "fullness" in the eye, but no pain. It normally occurs without cause, but can appear after a blunt trauma, or violent coughing, sneezing, or vomiting.

Treatment: Herbal eyewash may be used, but generally no treatment is necessary, even though this condition looks very painful.

STIES and CHALAZIA

Definition/Diagnosis: These infections of the eyelid can cause scratching of the cornea surface. Often the person thinks that something is in the eye when, in fact, one of these small pimples is forming. The sty is an infection along a hair follicle on the eyelid margin. The chalazion is an infection of an oil gland on the inner lid margin. The person will have redness, pain, and swelling along the edge of the upper or lower eyelid. At times the eye will be red with evidence of infection, or conjunctivitis. An eyelid may be swollen, without the pimple formation, when this problem first develops. There should not be extensive swelling around the eye. Generalized swelling around the eye in the absence of trauma could result from periorbital cellulitis which is a serious infection requiring more aggressive treatment.

Make sure a foreign body is not causing the symptoms. Check the eyes and eyelids. Confirm whether or not a pimple formation may be scratching the eye while blinking.

Treatment: Treat with warm compresses 20 minutes every two hours to cause the sty to come to a head. Also use herbal eyewash every two hours before the warm compresses. The red raspberry will help to dissolve and break up mucus congestion and build up. If it does not come to a head in two days, open the pimple with a needle and continue with the warm compresses and herbal eyewash.

MOTION SICKNESS

Treatment: Ginger root has proven to be effective for prevention and treatment of motion sickness, whether in a car or on a boat. Take either in the form of capsules, tincture or crystallized ginger.

NASAL CONGESTION

Nasal congestion is usually caused by an allergic reaction to pollen, dust, or other allergens. It may also be a viral or bacterial upper respiratory infection.

Treatment: Herbal snuff is effectively used to cleanse and disinfect the nose. Take immune enhancing herbs such as Goldenseal, echinacea, cat's claw or Immune Boost (see page 230).

Drink lots of fluids to prevent the mucus from becoming too thick. Thick mucus will not drain well and this tends to allow it to pack the sinus cavities with increasingly painful pressure. I define drinking a lot of fluids to be one gallon in 24 hours. And of course, you may as well make it herbal tea (red raspberry or peppermint are both good choices).

NOSE - Foreign Body in it

Foul drainage from one nostril is a tell-tale sign of a foreign body stuck in the nose. This is more common in children. Personally I've had to remove from the noses of kids raisins, peas and crayons.

Treatment: Have the person try to blow their nose to remove the foreign body. Don't permit violent nose-blowing. With an infant or small child a parent can gently puff into the child's' mouth while holding the other nostril closed to force the object out. You can spread the nostril open with hemostats stretching the nose open and with a flashlight attempt to see the foreign body. Using tweezers very gently grasp the object that you can directly see, and pull it out. Use good judgment and be cautious. If the foreign material is loose debris, like a capsule that broke in the persons mouth which was sneezed into the nostrils, it can best be irrigated out with a bulb or syringe. Place the bulb or syringe in the clear nostril and with the patient repeating an "eng" sound, flush water and hopefully debris out the opposite nostril.

After removing a foreign body, be sure to check the nostril again for anything additional. Do not try to push an object down the back of the persons throat as they might choke on it. If this is unavoidable, have the person face down and bend over to decrease the chance of choking. After pushing the object further into the nose and into the upper part of the pharynx (oral cavity), hopefully the victim can cough the object out. If you are going to use this technique be sure you are familiar with the sections on nose bleeds and the Heimlich maneuver. Don't probe your nose by yourself; you may push the object deeper or injure the nostril.

NOSEBLEEDS

If nose bleeding is caused from trauma to the nose, it is usually self limiting and easier to manage. Bleeding that started without trauma is generally more difficult to stop. Most bleeding is from small arteries located near the front of the nose partition, or nasal septum.

Treatment: The best treatment is direct pressure. Have the person pinch the fleshy part of the nose and place an ice pack on the back of the neck and sit quietly for ten minutes watching the clock. (It will seem like a very long time). This may cause a clot to form over the ruptured blood vessels. On releasing pressure, refrain from blowing the nose. If this fails administer a dropperful of cayenne tincture taken orally and continue to pinch the nose for an additional 10 minutes. Placing a piece of gauze between the upper lip and upper gum can stimulate a reflex helping the bleeding to stop.

If the bleeding continues, pack each bleeding nostril with a plug of sterile gauze or cotton dipped in water then dab in cayenne powder or tincture. It will burn a bit, but is safe and will stop the bleeding. Yarrow tincture on a cotton swap rubbed inside the nose can be effective. Take more cayenne or shepherd's purse internally. Be careful to leave one end of each plug outside so that it can be easily removed. Have the patient lie down with his head elevated and place a cold, wet towel across his face. If the bleeding is severe, have the patient sit up to prevent choking on the blood. This will also reduce the blood pressure in the nose. Continued bleeding can result in shock. This will in turn decrease the bleeding.

NOSE FRACTURE (Broken Nose)

Definition/Diagnosis: A direct blow causing a nasal fracture is associated with pain, swelling, and nasal bleeding. The pain is usually point tender, which means that a very light touch causes pain, indicating that a fracture has occurred at that location. While bleeding from trauma to the nose can initially be intense, it seldom lasts for more than a few minutes.

Treatment: Apply a cold compress, if available. Allow the patient to pinch their nose to reduce bleeding.

If the nose is laterally displaced (shoved to one side), push it back into place. More of these fractures have been treated by coaches on the playing field than by doctors. Don't be afraid, just do it. If it is a depressed fracture, a specialist will have to properly elevate the fragments. Rarely is a broken nose in need of being packed with gauze and this should be avoided as it will cause more pain.

Provide herbs for pain such as California poppy, Jamaican Dogwood, etc. as needed. CTR ointment and syrup (see page 224) can be used to speed healing and recovery.

SINUSITIS

Definition/Diagnosis: Sinusitis is the inflammation or infection of the sinuses (the air-filled cavities behind the nose and eyes). Symptoms are headache, sinus pain and tenderness, stuffiness, yellow mucus (which often drips down the back of the throat), temporary loss of smell, fatigue and sometimes fever. Often a sinus infection is preceded by a cold.

Treatment: (1) Put very hot, wet towels over your whole upper face 3 to 4 times daily. **(2)** Inhale steam (make a peppermint tea to inhale, then drink) **(3)** Practice saline irrigation. Mix 1/2 teaspoon salt in 8 ounces of warm water. Lean your head over the sink. Inhale the liquid through one nostril at a time while closing the other with an index finger. You may use a rubber bulb syringe or purchase a Neti Pot. **(4)** Use Herbal snuff 2 to 3 times daily (see page 229). **(5)** Drink plenty of fluids 12-14 cups per day. This will promote drainage and cut the mucus. Avoid ice cold drinks, anything containing caffeine or alcohol, which can be dehydrating. **(6)** Cut & chop Horseradish and/or Onions. The juices from these can open up the sinuses. Eating fresh horseradish, wasabi (Japanese horseradish) or dry mustard can open the sinuses. **(7)** Drinking carrot juice will also cut the mucus.

Chapter 7

HEADACHES

While this is an herbal manual, do not overlook the positive and profound benefits that can come through other natural therapies such as the chiropractic adjustment (spinal manipulation), massage therapy and CranioSacral Therapy. Each of these can be effective in both the acute or chronic headache.

POSSIBLE HEADACHE CAUSES

If Headache occurs:	Possible causes
On awakening	Tension Headache, pg. 118 Allergies, pg. 93 Sinusitis, pg. 113 Can also be due to low humidity.
Affecting the jaw muscles or temples.	See TMJ, pg. 193 Tension Headache, pg. 118
Each afternoon or evening; after hours of desk work; with sore neck and shoulders.	Tension Headache, pg. 118
On one side of the head.	Migraine Headache, pg. 117 Cluster Headaches, pg. 119
After a blow to the head.	Head Injuries, pg. 32
After exposure to chemicals (paint, varnish, insect spray, cigarette smoke).	Chemical Headache. Get into fresh air. Drink water to flush Out poisons. Take Colon

	Detox and Lung formula until symptoms subside.
With fever, runny nose, or sore throat.	Sinusitis, pg. 113 Flu, pg. 246 Sore Throat, pg. 177
With fever, stiff neck, nausea and vomiting.	Spinal Meningitis, pg. 171
With runny nose, watery eyes, and sneezing.	Allergies, pg 93
With fever and pain in the cheek or over the eyes.	Sinusitis, pg. 113
On morning when you drink less caffeine than usual.	Caffeine withdrawal headache. Cut back slowly but do get off of the caffeine.
Following a stressful event. Often after the stress is over.	Tension Headache, pg. 118
At the same time during menstrual cycle.	Menstrual problems, pg. 142
With new medication.	Drug allergy. Contact your pharmacist or prescribing doctor.
With severe eye pain.	Acute glaucoma. See doctor now!
Severe pain in children without trauma	Possible Tumor, if pain does not resolve within a day or two.

Most headaches respond very well to natural care. Some headaches may signal a life-threatening illness. If you experience any of the following symptoms call 911 or get to medical help as soon as possible.

1. A major exception may be the headache caused by bacterial meningitis. This is an infection within the lining of the brain. If the patient has symptoms characteristic of meningitis go to the emergency room immediately. Symptoms include; headache, stiff neck, high fever, sore throat, vomiting, and sensitivity to light. With an infant look for fever, poor muscle tone, a high-pitched cry and a bulging of the soft

spot (fontanel).

2. The headache is the worst of your life and came on very suddenly and severely. This could be a sign of an aneurysm rupturing or intracranial bleeding.

3. Your arms and legs on one side are weak, numb or paralyzed, or one side of your face appears droopy. You are unable to talk or express yourself clearly. These are signs of a stroke (see page 141).

4. Your headache grows steadily worse over time. You have repetitive vomiting. Seizures or convulsions. These symptoms can indicate a tumor.

DEHYDRATION HEADACHE

Definition/Diagnosis: Oh! I hate these. This headache results from not drinking enough fluids during physical activity. It is an early sign of dehydration (see page 148). The pain is felt on both sides of the head and is usually made worse when standing from a lying position.

Treatment: Rest and drink at least one to two quarts of water or rehydration solution. Follow instructions for dehydration.

MIGRAINE HEADACHE

Definition/Diagnosis: Often the term migraine is used for any severe headache, however it should be reserved for headaches that show specific patterns. The pain of a migraine is due to excessive dilation or contraction of blood vessels in the brain. A true migraine headache will involve only one side of the head and is often associated with nausea, vomiting and sensitivity to light. Walking or physical exertion will make the pain worse. About 15 percent of people with migraine headaches will experience an aura (flashing lights, distorted shapes and colors, blurred vision or other visual or even auditory apparitions) prior to the onset of the headache. Often migraines are triggered by food allergies or sensitivities, see Allergies page 93.

Treatment: Migraine headaches respond well to Headache Formula or Feverfew up to 4-5 dropperfuls every hour. Ginkgo, cayenne, chamomile and peppermint are also useful for these

...daches. If you are not a caffeine user, then 1-2 cups of strong offee, black tea or caffeinated soda at the onset of a migraine can arrest it. If you use caffeine regularly (coffee or soda), then caffeine will be ineffective as a treatment.

TENSION HEADACHES
Stress or Muscle Contraction Headache

Definition/Diagnosis: Of the many types of headaches, ninety percent are tension headaches. The pain is related to the muscles of the scalp and upper neck continuously contracting. These headaches can last from 30 minutes to many days. The headache is described as tight or vise-like and is felt on both sides of the head, but especially in the back of the head and upper neck. The pain is not made worse by physical activity. Photosensitivity (sensitive to bright light) may occur, but nausea and vomiting are not usually present.

Treatment: Massaging the back of the scalp, neck and upper back is very effective. Twin Tennis Ball Therapy (see page 263) and Relaxing meditation. Herbally, relaxing herbs such as chamomile, valerian, kava kava are useful. Combinations such as Nerve Calm (see page 232) can be used. Rub peppermint essential oil into the temples being careful not to get the oil into the eyes. An ice pack on the back of the neck can give relief.

ADDITIONAL TYPES of HEADACHES

Constipation is a major cause for headaches. Cleanse the colon with Colon Cleanse and Colon Detox (see page 254). Drink plenty of water as dehydration is a major cause of constipation.

Arthritis Headache: Pain at the back of the head or neck, made worse by movement; inflammation of joints and shoulder and/or neck muscles. Causes: degenerative osteoarthritis, post-traumatic arthritis.

Treatment: Take the herb Feverfew or Headache Formula (page 227). Treat arthritis with diet and herbal supplementation. See a good chiropractor.

Bilious Headache: Dull pain in forehead and throbbing temples. Usually caused by indigestion, overeating and lack of exercise.

Treatment: Cleanse the colon, see constipation. Follow the colon cleanse and colon detox programs.

Caffeine Headache: Throbbing pain caused by blood vessels that have dilated. Associated with caffeine withdrawal.

Treatment: Take in a small amount of caffeine, then begin to taper off caffeine completely. Yes, there is life without coffee and soda.

Cluster Headache: Severe, throbbing pain on one side of the head, flushing of the face, tearing of the eyes, nasal congestion. This headache occurs 1 to 3 times a day over a period of weeks or months and lasts from a few minutes to several hours each time. This type of headache usually results from stress, alcohol or smoking.

Treatment: Taking Ginkgo biloba or cayenne is useful. Headache formula is beneficial. Take care of the cause. Medical management may be necessary.

Exertion Headache: Generalized headache during or after physical exertion such as running or sex. This headache can even occur with passive exertion such as sneezing or coughing. This headache is usually seen in combination with a migraine or cluster headache. About 10 percent of these headaches can be related to organic diseases such as tumors or blood vessel malformation.

Treatment: Apply ice packs at the site of pain. Boost nutrition generally, see SuperNutrition page 217. Cleanse the channels of elimination (colon, liver, kidneys, lungs, skin) (see pages 254-259).

Eyestrain Headache: Usually bilateral, frontal pain due to eye muscle imbalance, uncorrected vision or astigmatism.

Treatment: Correct vision either through exercises such as the Bates Method or with corrective lenses.

Fever Headache: This headache develops with fever due to inflammation of blood vessels in the head during an infectious illness or infection.

Treatment: Treat the illness herbally as may be appropriate. Ice packs over the site of pain is helpful.

Hangover Headache: This migraine-like throbbing headache often is accompanied by nausea. Alcohol causes dehydration and dilation of the blood vessels in the brain.

Treatment: Drink plenty of pure water and fruit juices. Take liver detoxifying herbs such of oregon grape root, milk thistle and burdock root. Liver-Gallbladder formula (page 232) is useful.

Hunger Headache: By skipping meals, fasting or dieting too strictly, this headache can result due to low blood sugar, muscle tension and the rebound dilation of blood vessels. As the body begins to metabolize (burn) fats, toxins can be released causing the headache.

Treatment: Eat (duh). If weight loss is your objective, realize that going hungry will result in slowing your metabolism and is not an efficient way to lose weight long term.

Hypertension Headache: Dull, generalized pain affecting a large area of the head and aggravated by movement or exertion. This is accompanied by severely high blood pressure.

Treatment: Get the blood pressure under control.

Menstrual Headache: Migraine-like pain shortly before, during, or after menstruation, or at mid-cycle associated with ovulation. This is caused by fluctuating estrogen levels.

Treatment: Female balancing herbs, such as Black Cohosh (don't take if pregnant), Vitex, Angelica, Wild Yam, or a combination such as Female Balancing Formula (page 227).

Sinus Headache: Gnawing, nagging pain over the nasal and sinus areas often increase as the day goes by. Fever and discolored (non clear) mucus may be present. Sinus headaches are generally associated with allergies, infection, and/or nasal polyps.

Treatment: see sinusitis page 113.

TMJ (temporomandibular joint) Headache: Pain in the temple, above the ear or facial pain. The muscles on one side of the jaw are contracting stronger than the other, often resulting in a popping or clicking of the jaw. Neck or upper back and temple pain upon waking are often present. Stress is almost always a major issue. Malocclusion (a bad bite position), jaw clenching, gum chewing or bruxism (grinding teeth in sleep) are often seen.

Treatment: See TMJ page 193.

Temporal Headache: Jabbing, burning, boring pain in the temples or around the ear. Often aggravated by chewing, seen in weight loss and with eyesight problems. More common in people over 55. This headache is due to inflammation of the temporal arteries, appearing red and swollen around the temples.

Treatment: Cayenne (1/2 to 1 tsp. 3 times daily). This condition is rare and if untreated can result in stroke or blindness. Seek competent medical attention.

Trauma Headache: Dull, aching, stabbing and sharp or excruciating pain at the site of injury. If the headache is persistent and worsens with time and is accompanied by sleepiness, confusion, visual disturbance, nausea and/or vomiting, you must suspect a Subdural Hematoma (a blood clot within the brain or cranial vault) developing. Medical attention is necessary immediately.

Treatment: See head injury, page 32.

There are many, many more types of headaches. This short list will cover about 98% of those you are likely to encounter.

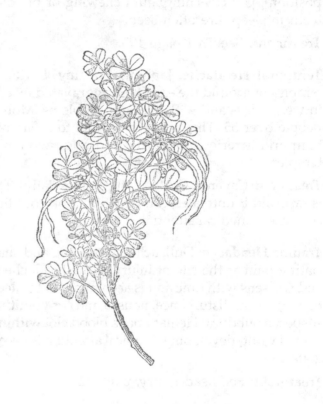

Chapter 8

SKIN & NAIL PROBLEMS

ABSCESS - Boil, Furnuncle

Definition/Diagnosis: An abscess is a pocket of pus (white blood cells), germs, and red blood cells that accumulate in a tissue, organ, or confined space in the body often resulting in infection. This is a protective mechanism of the body to prevent further spread of the germs. It is part of the body's natural immune response. Abscesses may be located internally or externally. The infected body part becomes swollen, inflamed and tender. Antibiotics can be ineffective in treating abscesses because the site is walled off and circulation and penetration through the blood supply is poor. Abscesses are very painful because of the pressure generated within them.

Treatment: Warm moist compresses can be effectively used to bring the abscess to the surface and to a head. Use blood cleansing herbs such as burdock, cayenne, dandelion root, Milk Thistle, red clover and yellow dock. Essiac tea and Western Botanicals' Blood Cleansing Formula can be effectively used. Apply a poultice of colon detox powder and immune boost tincture to draw out toxins. Once the abscess has broken out, clean thoroughly with soapy water and apply CTR ointment to the area of abscess until the skin returns to normal. Drink plenty of fluids, get plenty of bed rest. Take a complete nutritional supplement such as SuperNutrition 2-3 times daily. Boost the Immune System with echinacea, garlic, Goldenseal, cat's claw, or Astragalus.

An abscess may need to be cut open and drained surgically. The best anesthesia to use in this case is ice. Injecting an analgesic (pain killer) into the area will only cause more pain. Abscesses can be so painful that the person will often welcome the knife. Anything to relieve the pain. Spread of infection is unlikely if cleansed and treated properly.

ACNE

Acne is an inflammatory skin disorder resulting from the clogging of pores in the skin. Cleansing the blood and the liver are important. Often cleansing the colon and correcting constipation (our bodies should have 2-3 normal bowel movements each day, see "Constipation" page 51) Good nutritional habits must be adopted (See "The Health Building Diet," page 243). Wash afflicted areas with Castile soaps 2-3 times daily. No junk food or greasy foods. Double or triple SuperNutrition and Essiac Tea 2 oz. 2x daily and/or Liver-gallbladder Formula. Garlic taken orally destroys bacteria and enhances the immune system.

ATHLETE'S FOOT (Jock Itch, Foot fungus, etc.)

Definition/Diagnosis: Athlete's foot is a fungal infection that thrives in an environment of warmth and dampness. Symptoms include inflammation, burning, itching, scaling, cracking and blisters.

Treatment: If area is moist sprinkle with ginger root powder. Use CTR ointment, garlic oil, tea tree oil, or Pau d'Arco tincture applied directly to the area. Drinking Pau d'arco tea - 3 cups daily is advised. Olive leaf tincture or capsules 3 times daily is useful. A footbath of olive leaf and Pau d'arco tea with 20 drops of tea tree oil in a small tub of water for 15 minutes 3 times per day is effective.

BLISTERS

Prevention: It is important that you eliminate as many possible contributing factors to friction blisters as you can.

Make sure shoes fit properly. A shoe that is too tight causes pressure sores; one that is too loose results in friction blisters. Break in new shoes or boots gradually before your trip.

Wear a thin liner sock under a heavier one. Friction will occur between the socks rather than against your foot. Avoid prolonged wetness. It breaks down the skin, predisposing your feet to blisters. Keep your feet dry and use foot powder if necessary. A little cayenne powder, dry mustard or ginger powder will keep feet warm in the cold. Apply moleskin to sensitive areas where you may normally blister before you start hiking.

Hot Spots

Hot spots are sore, red areas of irritation which, if allowed to progress, develop into blisters.

Treatment of hot spots:

1. Take a rectangular piece of moleskin (moleskin is soft cotton flannel with adhesive on the back), or molefoam, which is thicker and quite a bit more protective than moleskin, and cut an oval-shaped hole in the middle(like a donut) the size of the hot spot.

2. Center this over the hot spot and secure it in place, making sure that the sticky surface is not on the irritated skin. The moleskin acts as a buffer against further rubbing.

3. Apply Complete Tissue Repair Ointment (see page 224) to the hot spot. It will soothe and begin healing the area. Do not put the CTR on before the moleskin is in place.

4. Reinforce the mole skin with tape or a piece of non-woven adhesive knit dressing.

Blister Treatment:

- If the blister is small and still intact, the unbroken skin covering a blister is the best protection against infection. Place a piece of moleskin with a donut style hole cut slightly larger than the blister over the site. The moleskin or molefoam should be thick enough to keep the shoe from rubbing the blister. Use several layers if necessary.

- If the blister is larger or if the blister has broken, puncture it with a clean needle or safety pin at its base, and massage out the fluid. Sterilize the needle with a match. The blister fluid contains inflammatory juices that can delay healing.

- Trim away any loose skin from the bubble with scissors.

- Wash the area gently with soap and water, then apply Herbal Anti-Septic tincture or Complete Tissue Repair Ointment and cover with a sterile dressing. Use freshly-picked Plantain or Mullein leaves in your shoes to prevent blisters. Use a plantain poultice if blister develops. Use Immune Boost to prevent infection. Moleskin or Spenco 2nd skin are good commercial products that can be used especially if you are hiking or need to keep walking. Cut a donut style hole as described above. Cover the blister with CTR ointment after you place the moleskin on. Cover the moleskin hole and ointment covered blister-wound with sterile gauze. If no moleskin or molefoam is available, place a piece of tape over the hot spot where a blister is beginning to form. Duct tape works good. You can also use a piece of cloth or other material.

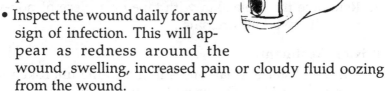

- Inspect the wound daily for any sign of infection. This will appear as redness around the wound, swelling, increased pain or cloudy fluid oozing from the wound.

ECZEMA

Definition/Diagnosis: There are many steroid based medicines that in essence drive the problem deeper back into the body. As with most skin conditions, this is a toxicity or cleansing issue. If the body is not able to eliminate toxins adequately through the normal channels of elimination (the bowel, lungs, liver, kidney) then it will come out through the skin causing irritation, blistering, itching etc. Eczema is not an infection, but the blisters or rash if scratched or rubbed persistently can become infected.

Treatment: First you must cleanse the colon. Use enough colon cleanse, see page 222, to insure you have 2 to 3 normal bowel movements daily. Then cleanse the liver with the Liver Flush and begin taking liver and blood cleansing herbs such as Essiac Tea, Milk Thistle, Oregon Grape root, Chickweed, or Dandelion. You may treat the skin with CTR Ointment applied to the area during the day. Black Ointment or Colon Detox/Immune Boost poultice applied at night, especially if there are blisters that are weepy. Chickweed tea used as a fomentation helps to detoxify

EDEMA

Definition/Diagnosis: Edema or swelling of the tissues is a symptom, not a disease itself. Edema can be brought on from as diverse things as congestive heart failure to eating too much salt in the diet the night before. If swelling of the skin is the only symptom you are experiencing, often flushing the kidneys will be enough to resolve the issue. This can be done by simply drinking plenty of water, but as long as you're drinking water, you may as well drink a mild herbal tea. Good diuretic herbs such as corn silk (the stringy tassels you peel off whole ears of corn), uva ursi or parsley all are very effective.

One complication of simple edema occurs with swollen fingers and the wearing of rings. The swelling of fingers with a tight ring can cut off the circulation causing extreme pain that can even result in the loss of the finger. Excess fluid can be milked out of the finger and with the use of a string or thread, the finger can be narrowed in thickness to slide the ring off as illustrated at right.

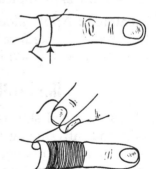

FUNGAL INFECTIONS
Groin, Arm Pit, Scrotum, Rectum, Under Breasts, Ringworm

Treatment: Tea tree/Jojoba oil (10% tea tree/ 90% Jojoba) over affected area. Also garlic oil over affected area. Take Black Walnut tincture 1-2 dropperfuls 3 times daily. Drink 3 cups of Pau d'arco tea daily.

FUNGUS (under finger and toe nails)

Definition/Diagnosis: This pernicious problem can be very difficult to manage and get under control. It requires persistence and dedication. There are now drugs that can be taken orally to fight this fungal infection. However they come at a high cost to the liver.

Treatment: Take Nettle Tincture internally, 1-2 dropperfuls 3 times daily. Externally, apply Nettle Tincture or soak in Nettle Tea. Also file the outer layer of the nail off to expose the fungal infection. Use tea tree oil directly on nails. This must be done 3-4 times per week for many months or the life of the nail. Soak your feet or hands in a tea made of pau d'arco and Goldenseal. Soak for 15 minutes twice daily. The enzyme protease made into a paste and used topically twice daily is effective.

HIVES

Definition/Diagnosis: Hives are the result of a severe allergic reaction. Commonly called welts, these raised red blotches develop rapidly and frequently have a red border around a clearer skin area in the center, sometimes referred to as an "annular lesion". As these can and do appear over large surfaces of the skin, topical treatment is largely ineffective.

Treatment: Apply aloe vera gel to the affected areas. Boost the immune system response with Immune Boost, echinacea or cat's claw. Use Willard's water as a topical wash.

IMPETIGO (Bacterial skin rash)

This superficial skin rash is often caused by scratching the skin and introducing bacteria from the fingernails. Often it will occur in conjunction with an unrelated rash. The normal appearance of impetigo is reddish areas around pus filled blisters, which are frequently crusty and scabbed. The lesions spread rapidly over a few days time. The skin is generally not swollen underneath the lesions. It is most commonly found around the nose and on the buttocks. It spreads rapidly from scratching and can spread to anywhere on the body. Early lesions should be cleansed with soapy water and herbal anti-septic tincture.

Treatment: Treat the patient with Immune Boost and/or Anti-

Plague formula 4-6 times daily. Avoid scratching the area, which can lead to spreading and infection. Wash with Antiseptic wash 2 to 3 times daily.

ITCH

Definition/Diagnosis: The itch sensation is transmitted by pain fibers, so all pain herbs can be used to alleviate the itch sensation. Itch usually is an indication of something being awry and possibly requiring specific treatment. The most common causes are local allergic reactions, such as poisonous plants (page 158), fungal infections(see page 127), and insect bites (see page 183). Avoid further contact with the offending substances. Avoid applying heat to an itchy area. This makes it worse. Avoid scratching or rubbing, this also increases the reaction. If weeping blisters have formed, apply wet soaks with a clean cloth or gauze. A solution of epsom salts or even regular table salt will help. Apple Cider Vinegar diluted to 50% with distilled (or at least purified) water applied to the area will relieve itching. Be sure to buy real apple cider vinegar and don't make the mistake I once did by buying apple cider "flavored" vinegar.

NAILS - Ingrown

This painful infection along the edge of a nail can, at times, be relieved with soaking the foot in warm water (with epsom salts, or mullein tea. There are several things you can do to speed the healing. First take a piece of strong tape (such as first aid waterproof tape) and tape it next to the inflamed skin edge (next to - but not touching the nail). The tape is fastened tightly to this skin edge with gentle, but firm pressure. Next run the tape under the toe so that the skin edge is being pulled away from the nail. This can relieve the pressure.

Another method is to shave the top of the nail by scraping it with a sharp blade until it is thin enough that it buckles upwards. This "breaks the arch" of the nail and allows the ingrown edge to be forced out of the inflamed groove along the side. Use either of these techniques at the first sign of irritation rather than waiting for an infection to develop.

NAILS - Subungual Hematoma

This is blood under a fingernail or toenail. It is generally caused by trauma to the nail (smashing it or dropping something heavy on it). The accumulation of blood under the nail can create tremendous pressure and be very painful. Relieve this pressure by twirling the sharp point of a blade (using the lightest pressure possible) until a hole is drilled through and the blood can drain. Soak in cool water to promote the drainage of this blood. Herbal pain formula can be used if necessary. Apply with CTR ointment and cover with a bandaid.

POISON OAK, IVY & SUMAC (Contact dermatitis)

Wash the area with soap and cold water working up a thick lather rinsing several times. Do not scrub with a brush as this can cut in to the skin spreading the oils into the blood. Make sure the affected clothing is removed. Often the antidote to these irritants can be found within 10-20 yards of the plant. (looks for some Hounds Tongue or Jewelweed to rub on affected area). A strong decoction of Manzanita leaves acts as a strong astringent and is used externally on the skin.

If itching and burning already appear, wash the affected areas gently with soap and cold water, and pat on one of the remedies below. Avoid scratching, rubbing or touching the effected areas.

Remedy: *Mix 2 tablespoons each of Gindella (Jewelweed, this is used in many commercial preparations under the name 2-methoxy-1, 4-naphthoquinone) and comfrey leaf*

1/4 cup Apple Cider Vinegar

3 drops peppermint essential oil

1/2 teaspoon salt

Apply to affected areas.

Paste: *1/8 cup of above remedy*

1/8 cup distilled water

1/4 cup Colon Detox powder

Apply as you would a poultice

Bath: *4 drops each of peppermint and lavender essential oils*

4 cups of ground or powdered oats

1 cup of Epsom salt

Use Immune Boost internally as you would an infection. One to two dropperfuls 3-4 times daily. Immune boost applied directly to eruptions is known to take the itch away immediately as does plantain either in tea, poultice or tincture form.

Symptoms that may warrant medical attention include an extensive rash that covers more than half of the body; extreme swelling and redness, and fever. Consult a healthcare provider if eruptions occur near the eyes, mouth or genitals.

RASHES and SKIN ERUPTIONS

Most rashes can be traced to coming in contact with an irritant that a person is allergic to such as poison oak/ivy or sumac, or a new washing detergent, or because of food allergies. First identify if the patient has come in contact with an irritant like poison oak or a new detergent. If so refer to Poison Oak (page 130). There are seven foods which are responsible for most of the cases of atopic dermatitis (rashes that are not from contacting an irritant). Cows Milk, eggs and peanuts top the list for causing rash and eczema, followed by fish (particularly cod and catfish), wheat, soybeans and cashews. Chocolate, corn, pork and beef have also been implicated in skin rashes. As well as pesticides, herbicides and other poisons that are sprayed on produce.

Treatment: Eliminate any suspect food from your diet for at least 10 days before you carefully re-introduce any of them.

A soothing wash made of Calendula, chamomile, elder flower and tea tree oil can be used externally. Make a strong tea of these herbs and add 5-10 drops of tea tree oil per cup of tea/ wash. Take Plantain Tincture 1-2 dropperfuls 3 times daily

Yarrow Tincture 1-2 dropperfuls 3 times daily.

CTR Ointment over the effected area 3 times daily. Essiac tea used daily is beneficial for chronic cases. A fomentation made of the following herbs will reduce inflammation:

6 parts Oak bark

3 parts Mullein

1 part Lobelia

6 parts Comfrey

Use one ounce of herb combination of 2 cups of water. Reduce over heat to 1/2 cup. Use as a fomentation on the areas of the rash. BioSET Allergy Elimination treatments should also be explored.

RASH- DIAPER

Definition/Diagnosis: While not a first aid emergency, this condition if left without adequate treatment can blister and bleed causing much distress to infant and parent. First use the CTR ointment, see page 224. Slippery Elm powder or Colon Detox powder over the area can also be used. Expose the area to sunlight. Mother, if nursing, should take Immune Boost tincture.

ULCERS - decubitus ulcers, bedsores, pressure sores

Definition/Diagnosis: Bedsores or pressure sores are deep ulcers that form when pressure is exerted over bony areas of the body, restricting circulation and leading to the death of cells in the overlying tissue.

Treatment: CTR ointment or comfrey ointment should be packed. Make sure the bowels move at least 1-2 times per day. Eat a healthy diet (see page 243).

WARTS

Garlic oil is an effective solution. The milky exudate from purslane is known as a wart remover. Massage into the wart area several times daily. A fresh slice of garlic held in place over a wart is effective, however because of the sulfur in garlic, it can burn the skin raising a blister.

Chapter 9

WOMEN'S HEALTH

CYSTITIS/URINARY TRACT INFECTIONS

Definition/Diagnosis: The urge to urinate frequently, burning with urination, only small amounts being voided, and pain in the lowest area of the abdomen is classic with a bladder infection. Often the patient will have a fever, chills and achy muscles. The urine can become cloudy or even bloody (a slight reddish or orange to brownish tint to the urine). If the urine is cloudy without the other symptoms, it does not mean they have a urinary tract infection (UTI). Infection can extend to the kidney with the resultant lower back and flank pain (in the back along the sides below the ribs - sometimes one side, often both). Bladder infections are more common in women but men are not exempt.

There are 14 factors that can contribute to cystitis or urinary tract infections.

1. Hygiene - wiping back to front, instead of front to back. Irritating chemicals from commercial douches, and swimming pool chemicals can lead to UTI's.
2. Sexual Intercourse or "Honeymoon Cystitis" - insure cleanliness and urinating before and after sexual intercourse.
3. Contraceptive Devices - Using a diaphragm that may be too large, contraceptive jelly can provide a medium for bacteria to get from vagina to urethra.
4. Tampons - these can often introduce foreign material and chemicals leaving the vagina vulnerable to bacterial over-

growth which can travel to the urethra.

5. Antibiotics - the use of antibiotics as a treatment for cystitis or other infections can create an environment where bacteria can flourish. Antibiotics do kill bacteria, but at a very high price: weakening your immune system. Antibiotics destroy good and bad bacteria alike. Good bacteria are vital to health. By taking antibiotics you become more vulnerable to chronic, recurring cystitis.

6. Inadequate Fluid Intake - Drink plenty of fluids and urinate at the first urge rather than "holding it".

7. Diet - Foods and beverages that are too spicy or acidic can irritate the bladder making it more susceptible to infection. Coffee and alcohol are the worst acidic offenders. Acidic foods include dairy products, red meat, tomatoes, red grapes, potatoes and strawberries.

8. Chronic Constipation - this results in toxins building up in the intestinal tract impairing immune function, making you more susceptible to infection.

9. Uterine Prolapse - this can be aggravated by constipation resulting in incomplete emptying of the bladder. Stagnant urine creates an ideal climate for bacteria overgrowth.

10. Hormonal Changes - menopausal women are more prone due to decreasing estrogen levels. Bacteria are more inclined to adhere to the bladder lining and vaginal walls with low estrogen levels. The vagina also can become dry making infection more likely.

11. Underactive Thyroid - this can result in a weakened immune system. Estrogen inhibits thyroid secretion.

12. Acidic Urine - This is related to an acidic diet and stress.

13. Energy Blockages - underclothing that is too tight, not urinating when the bladder is full, chronic stress, anxiety, tense muscle can all block energy flow to the body.

14. Unexpressed Anger or Resentment - this can lead to chronic cystitis.

Treatment: Use Kidney Bladder Formula and Tea (see page 230). Make and drink one gallon of Kidney-Bladder Tea in 24 hours. Add one dropperful of Kidney-Bladder tincture to each cup of tea. These formulae contain herbs such as juni-

per, parsley, uva ursi, corn silk etc. Cranberry juice can also
be of benefit (it seems to making the lining of the bladder slippery preventing the bacteria from adhering to the walls of
the bladder. The more you drink, the more you are flushing
out and washing away the infection. The herbs in these formulae work very effectively. But only if you use them. A few
sips or cups a day will not be enough.

Contrasting sitz baths can relieve cystitis pain and improve
circulation in the pelvic area. To prepare the baths, find two
basins or tubs that you can sit in comfortably. Fill one with hot
water to about the level of your navel, and the other with cold
water to the same level. Soak first in the hot bath for 3 to 5
minutes; then in the cold water for 30 seconds. Repeat three
times, finishing with the cold water. Do this once or twice daily.
Alternating hot and cold packs can be substituted.

BREASTS (Mastitis)
Sore, Swollen, Infected, Cracked Nipples

Definition/Diagnosis: This results when a milk duct become
clogged in the nursing mother. The breast swells, is hot and
very tender. Mastitis occurs with a nursing mother. Be very
suspicious of an infection if you are not nursing. Be aware of
the signs and symptoms of breast cancer.

Treatment: Immune Boost Formula 1-2 dropperfuls 5-6 times
daily. Use a hot fomentation of Mullein and shepherd's Purse
over the affected breast 3-5 times daily. The baby should be
nursed from different angles so that all of the milk ducts are
opened and utilized. Use Marshmallow root, SuperNutrition,
Horsetail and Nettle to enrich milk which will increase the milk
flow unclogging any ducts. CTR Ointment applied to affected
breast. Sage for drying up milk when mother is ready to quit
nursing. Therapeutic ultrasound can be used by an
expereinced practitioner.

CHILDBIRTH

Childbirth should not be viewed as an emergency procedure
even though there may be some anxiety or trepidation experienced when childbirth is imminent. Childbirth is a natural
and normal process. Never try to hurry or force the birth.
Let nature take its course. Make sure the area where the baby

is to be born is as clean as possible and any instruments have been sterilized by boiling or immersing in rubbing alcohol. Also, those assisting must wash hands thoroughly with soap (If possible).

Supplies to have on hand:

- 2 to 4 receiving blankets
- 2 towels
- 2 quart bowl (for placenta)
- A large plastic garbage bag (unused, of course)
- A light weight blanket (placed over the garbage bag for mom to lie on)
- Scissors (to cut the cord)
- Shoe string or dental floss (to tie the cord off)
- Bulb Syringe - for cleaning the baby's airway

During the birthing process, try to remain calm and reassuring to the mother. Remember, she is the one doing most of the work; your job is that of an assistant. Most complications during delivery occur when nature is interfered with so never interfere with the natural birthing process.

Encourage the mother to use the following positions:

- Hands & knees with a pillow between the lower legs
- Squatting over a pillow
- Side lying with the head propped
- No back lying. This results in a decreased blood supply to the baby which increases the risk of distress and could result with a depressed baby at birth.

When the baby starts to move down the birth canal, have the mother get in a comfortable position on a soft, yet firm surface (bedding or towels if available). As the baby's head begins to emerge, assist the mother by supporting the perineum (the area between the vaginal opening and anus) with a wash cloth in one hand to prevent the skin from tearing. With the other hand support the baby's head as it emerges. NEVER pull on the baby's head in order to speed up the delivery, but wait for the next contraction and mother's pushing action to facilitate the baby's birth. Support the emerging baby at the same level as the mother. Support the baby's head as it turns within the birth canal. As the head emerges, check to see if the umbilical cord is wrapped around the baby's neck. If it is, gently slip it over the baby's head. Do not hurry to cut the cord. Allow the baby to glide out supporting the child with a wash cloth - newborn babies are slippery so be careful.

When completely delivered, check for breathing in the baby. Clean debris from the mouth with a bulb syringe (or a finger-sweep will do) only if the child is not breathing. The baby should be held with his face down or to the side to permit sneezing and coughing to get out any mucus that may be in the nose or throat. If the baby is blue or pale and doesn't cry or breathe within one minute gently rub the baby's back up and down with a receiving blanket to stimulate the baby. If the child is unresponsive gently administer artificial respiration by gently blowing puffs of air by mouth to mouth/nose artificial respiration. Talk to the baby and be gentle.

If the umbilical cord is long enough, place the baby on the mothers chest and tummy. Place a receiving blanket and towel over the baby to absorb moisture. Allow the mothers body heat to comfort and keep the baby warm. Allow the baby and the mother to try to nurse (Nursing helps the uterus contract to help expel the placenta). If the umbilical cord is not long enough, place the baby in the space between the mother's thighs (with the baby's head slightly lowered and turned to the side) until the umbilical cord is cut. Be sure the baby is covered for warmth.

The placenta will follow the baby, usually in a few minutes, sometimes after many hours. If the woman isn't bleeding, don't do anything to hasten the delivery of the placenta. If there is some bleeding or cramping, stimulate the mothers nipples. This will cause the uterus to contract. Having the infant nurse can accomplish this. Giving the mother Blue Cohosh and/or Angelica root can also cause uterine contractions. Never pull on the cord to deliver the placenta. You will be able to detect when the placenta separates from the wall of the uterus when: cramping and contractions begin again, you observe a gush of blood, the cord lengthens and the mother pushes again.

After the placenta/after birth is expelled, make sure the mother isn't bleeding excessively. Rub the mothers tummy between the navel and the pubic bone until you feel a hard ball the size of a grapefruit. Normally the total amount of blood loss should not exceed two cups. The suckling of the baby at the breast will minimize blood loss. Manual compression of the uterus by holding it firmly together between two hands may be necessary in an emergency. Also Cayenne, Shepherd's Purse (use only if the uterus feels firm) or Mistletoe can be administered orally in powdered or tincture form to stop a hemorrhage. Horsetail tea is also helpful. Keep both mother and baby warm and resting. Give the mother 8 ounces or more of juice or other fluids.

The cord should not be dealt with until the placenta is delivered and the mother is out of danger, unless it is a short cord and won't allow for the mother to nurse. Make sure it has stopped pulsating and then tie a sterile string around the umbilical cord about 3-4 inches from the baby. Tie a second string around the umbilical cord about 3 inches away from the first one. Shoestring can be used. Immerse scissors or knife in boiling water or clean with alcohol. Cut the umbilical cord between the two ties with a sterile knife or scissors.

While the mother rests, the baby can be dressed or wrapped in a blanket to be kept warm. The natural grease or white material should not be washed off the baby's body as it is a protective coating for the baby's skin. Of course, any blood or debris should be gently wiped away. Do nothing to the baby's eyes, ears and nose.

Urgent skills may be necessary for the following:

- Partial separation of the placenta with more blood loss
- Baby is not coming around (not breathing)
- A shoulder is stuck
- Cord is tight around the neck.
- Birth is breach
- Limb presentation

Notify the mother's physician or midwife and transport the mother and child as necessary.

Key points to remember:

- Have something soft for the mother to be on.
- Have something soft for the baby to land on.
- Have towels and blankets for warmth.
- Support the perineum.

- Help the baby make the U-turn.
- Stimulate the baby if needed after one minute.
- Nurse as soon as the baby is ready.
- The birth process is natural and normal. Just let it happen.

When all is normal (and you should expect it to be) - enjoy the process of witnessing the birth of a new life.

ENDOMETRIOSIS

Definition/Diagnosis: small patches of uterine lining tissue (called endometrium) migrate to and implant themselves in other parts of the pelvic areas such as the ovaries, fallopian tubes, uterine muscles, colon, bladder and sides of the pelvic cavity. These endometrial implants (called endometriomas) contain brown blood debris and upon rupturing, they spill into the pelvic cavity creating irritation and inflammation. During menstruation, these endometriomas swell with blood and bleed, after which scar tissue forms in the injured location leading to a buildup of dense tissue adhesions. The pain and inflammation can be debilitating. Causes of endometriosis include:

1. Estrogen Dominance - This is an excess of estrogen relative to progesterone. Estrogen dominance is behind many women's health conditions including PMS. Symptoms such as bloating, weight gain, headaches, and backache are common with excess estrogen. Estrogen dominance can be created by eating foods high in estrogen (animal products - meat, dairy, eggs). Also herbicides, pesticides and the by-products of plastics manufacture can mimic estrogen once they enter the body. Chronic constipation or toxic buildup in the intestines cause excess estrogen to be reabsorbed by the body instead of being eliminated. Chronic stress, underactive thyroid gland and perimenopause (the 10 to 15 years before menopause) can all create estrogen dominance.

2. Early Onset of Menses and Delayed First Pregnancy

3. Underactive Thyroid Gland

4. Exposure to Environmental Estrogens - chemicals, animal products.

5. Weakened Immunity

6. Candidiasis - chronic yeast infections suppress the immune system which can lead to lead to endometriosis. Women with endometriosis should also follow anti-candida therapies.

7. Stressful emotional Patterns - often seen in women with demanding careers who may feel that their emotional selves are not being nurtured.

Treatment: Epsom Salt Bath: Add up to a quart of Epsom salt (magnesium sulfate) to a bathtub of hot water. Stir until the crystals dissolve, then immerse yourself up to your ears and soak for at least 20 minutes. After drying yourself, lie down on a towel on a bed for another 20 minutes. Epsom salt deeply relaxes muscles, and releases emotions, thoughts, and stress associated with tight, contracted muscles. Even after you have dried yourself, the Epsom salt is still working, which is why the post-bath relaxation period is important.

Castor Oil packs are used for relief of menstrual cramps, or a joints to relieve pain. To prepare a castor oil pack, lightly heat enough castor oil to thoroughly wet but not soak a 10" x 12" flannel cloth. Immerse the flannel in the hot oil, then fold to make three to four layers and place against the skin. (Castor oil helps to draw out toxins, release tension, and improve blood circulation, especially in the abdomen). Cover the flannel with clear plastic wrap (saran wrap) to keep towels from getting "goopy". Wrap a heating pad or hot water bottle in a towel and place this over the pack, then cover the pack and the bottle with another towel to retain the heat. Keep in place for one to two hours (a good time to watch a video). Following the treatment, the oil-soaked flannel may be wrapped in plastic or put in a zip lock bag and stored in the refrigerator for later use. After the flannel has been used 20 times, discard it.

Herbal formulae such a the female balancing formula (page 227) or effective. Wild yam and Chaste Tree (vitex) regulate hormone balance. Hawthorn berry is specific for endometriosis (1/4 tsp. twice daily). Flaxseed oil or another form of essential fatty acids is important (4 tsp. daily).

FIBROIDS

Definition/Diagnosis: Uterine fibroids are benign fibrous tumors of the uterus. Fibroids are firm lumps that usually occur in groups. They can range in size from microscopic to as big as a basketball. They can be very fast growing and result in severe lower abdominal pain. Excessive menstrual bleeding, miscarriages, anemia, weakness and dizziness, a feeling of fullness and pressure in the lower abdomen, bleeding between periods, increased menstrual cramps, lumps in the abdomen, and a chronic mucus discharge are common. Fibroids can cause constipation, urinary urgency, recurrent bladder infections. Conventional medical treatment is hysterectomy, however natural therapies have proven to be very effective without sacrificing the uterus. Fibroids are believed to be caused by hormonal imbalance, with an excess of estrogen and a deficiency of progesterone. See estrogen dominance on page 139. Estrogen dominance (too much estrogen in relation to progesterone) can be created by both an excess of estrogen and a deficiency of progesterone. Since hormones are 'deactivated' by the liver before they are eliminated, any liver congestion will lead to raised levels of circulating estrogen and thus aggravate fibroid growth. Too much estrogen may be caused by 1) foods that have hormones added to them such as commercial meat, milk, eggs, and dairy products 2) herbs that have an estrogenic effect in the body, such as licorice, black cohosh, and damiana 3) birth control pills that have high levels of estrogen 4) environmental toxins that mimic the actions of estrogen (the largest source is pesticides) 5) exposure to radiation, which increases estrogen levels in the blood 6) chronic constipation, which interferes with the body's ability to eliminate estrogen properly; estrogen then builds up in the colon and can be reabsorbed by the body 7) synthetic estrogen supplements as a part of a hormone replacement therapy for menopausal symptoms. Too little progesterone may be caused by; 1) an underactive thyroid gland 2) chronic stress 3) frequent anovulatory cycles (menstruation without ovulation).

Treatment: Various natural progesterone creams (1/4 to 1/ 2 tsp. daily) can be effective. Shepherd's purse taken only during menstruation (15 drops every 15 minutes until bleeding subsides). An herbal tea made from yucca, chaparral and chastetree berry (3 cups daily) is known to reduce fibroid size. Female Balancing formula (2-3 dropperfuls 3 times daily, page 227) has been very effective in stopping the bleeding and shrinking fibroids. Diet is very important (see health promoting diet, page 243). Nutritional support such as SuperNutrition (page 217) can be invaluable. Essential fatty acids (EFA's) such a flaxseed oil (4 tsp. daily), Evening primrose oil, or cod liver oil can be substituted. Chastetree berry, wild yam and dong quai (angelica senenses) are valuable herbal aids.

Castor oil packs (see page 140) or a Bentonite clay poultice over the uterine area can provide effective relief.

MENSTRUAL PROBLEMS

Dysmenorrhea - Pain and cramping during menstruation is classified as either primary or secondary Dysmenorrhea. Primary Dysmenorrhea occurs during the ovulatory cycle and is caused by excess production of prostaglandins (chemicals which cause the uterus to contract). In secondary dysmenorrhea menstural pain and cramping is secondary to an underlying factor such as endometriosis, pelvic inflammatory disease or fibroids. Causes can include hormonal imbalance, fluid retention, food sensitivities or allergies, liver toxicity, bladder infection, lack of exercise, poor circulation, stress, Intrauterine devices (IUDs), or vaginal yeast infections.

Treatment: Treat the underlying causes with diet, detoxification programs, and castor oil pack, hot water bottle over the uterus and herbal supplementation. Chastetree berry, wild yam, black cohosh, dong quai (Angelica sinensis), or the female balancing formula. Red raspberry tea should be taken daily (3 cups). As with most female or hormonal problems, therapies should be continued for months to achieve optimal results. For some it may take as long as 6 or 8 months of diligent self care before significant results are obtained. Be patient and hang in there. The alternative is to keep what you've got. Use pain formula (page 233) as needed. Massage cinnamon leaf essential oil to abdomen. Hot water bottle over uterus with ice pack on forehead or back of neck. Take Colon Cleanse (page 222) for constipation.

Menorrhagia - Excessive bleeding during menstruation

means that your period is too heavy, flows too fast, or the bleeding is moderate but persists for too long. A common cause is estrogen dominance. In addition to estrogen dominance, other physiological factors can produce heavy bleeding, such as endometriosis, fibroids, ovarian cysts, cervical cancer, thyroid dysfunction, pregnancy complications or miscarriage, or IUDs.

Treatment: Herbal support such as Shepherd's purse (15 drops every 15 minutes until bleeding subsides), natural progesterone (wild yam cream), castor oil packs, flaxseed oil (EFAs), dietary changes, and psychological counseling if necessary.

PMS - Premenstrual syndrome is characterized by bloating, cramping, achiness, headaches, short temper, irritability, sudden mood swings, depression, frustration, breast tenderness, crying spells, and abdominal discomfort occurring one to two days before a woman's period to the onset of bleeding. PMS has been classified into four basic types, PMS-A (for anxiety), PMS-C (for cravings), PMS-D (for depression) and PMS-H (for hyperhydration). PMS can have many causes (usually a combination of several) including; poor diet, estrogen dominance, underactive thyroid gland, exhausted adrenal glands, Candida albicans overgrowth, parasites, nutritional deficiencies, food sensitivities or allergies, environmental sensitivities, mercury dental filling, stress, sleep disorders, Caffeine, lack of sunlight, lack of exercise, and unresolved physical or sexual abuse.

Treatment: A multiple approach usually works best, combining dietary changes, herbal medicines,(an all-purpose PMS herb is chastetree berry (*Vitex agnus-castus*), female balancing herbs, liver detoxification, probiotics (acidophilus, bifidophilus, etc.), castor oil packs, natural progesterone therapy, and massage therapy (including acupressure and foot reflexology). Fish oils and flaxseed oils can offer relief from cramps (6 grams daily). Look into BioSET treatments for resolution.

MISCARRIAGE - Ectopic Pregnancy

Definition/Diagnosis: About 10-15% of pregnancies result in a spontaneous abortion or miscarriage. As long as everything passes, "a complete abortion", the bleeding and the pain will stop and the uterus will shrink back to its normal size. When the patient is threatening miscarriage give her a tea made of 3 parts false unicorn and 1 part lobelia. This will facilitate the miscarriage or prevent it from happening, which ever is appropriate for the fetus. The body is designed to reject an non-viable fetus. If all of the placental tissue did not come out and bleeding continues a surgeons care may be required. Use shepherd's purse to stop and control the bleeding. Apply pressure to the uterus is necessary. Use herbs for pain as necessary.

In an ectopic pregnancy (the fetus is outside of the uterus - usually stuck in a fallopian or uterine tube), spotting and cramping usually begin shortly after the first period is missed. Rupture of the uterine tube usually occurs at 6 to 8 weeks of pregnancy, while rupture of the outside of the uterine tube, but not in the uterus, occurs at 12 to 16 weeks. The rupture causes massive blood loss with a rapid onset of shock and death when it occurs. If a women experiences spotting and cramping lasting more than 24 hours, this could be a surgical emergency. If you are not sure she is pregnant, don't bet with her life. Get her to the emergency room immediately.

OVARIAN CYSTS

Definition/Diagnosis: Ovarian cysts develop on or in an ovary at any age between puberty and menopause. Often there are no symptoms but if the growth is large the ovary can become twisted or there can be abnormal hormone production. Other symptoms can include: Abdominal fullness or heaviness, pressure on the rectum or bladder, irregularities in the menstrual cycle, pelvic pain shortly before the onset or end of menstruation, pelvic pain during intercourse, nausea, vomiting, or breast tenderness. Conventional medical treatment is surgery, however in many cases conservative care is preferable. Causes include hormonal imbalance, hypothyroidism, poor diet, genetic predisposition, cigarette smoking, and psychological or emotional influences.

Treatment: Sitz baths are effective for treating painful ovaries (see page 135). Herbally the Turska Formula has been used to move blood, tumors and masses. This tincture is made from poke root, monkshood, gelsemium and bryonia. Take five drops daily. Balancing the hormones through diet, relieving constipation, castor oil packs, and dietary changes are important considerations.

UTERUS (Disorders, Prolapse)

Hemorrhages - Shepherd's Purse, Horsetail or Yarrow Tincture 1-2 dropperfuls 3 times daily. Female Balancing Formula 1-2 dropperfuls 3 times daily to normalize periods. Drink Red Raspberry Tea daily.

Prolapse - Empty colon with luke warm enema. Massage abdominal area with Shepherd's Purse Tincture starting from the vagina working upward. Use a slant board regularly. A vaginal pessary (see vaginits for pessary recipe) with female and astringent herbs. See a midwife or chiropractor who can adjust the uterus.

VAGINITIS

Definition/Diagnosis: This infection or inflammation of the vagina or vulva is hallmarked by uncomfortable itching and pain (often worse on urination and during sexual intercourse). It is caused by a variety of factors including candida (yeast) overgrowth, parasites, hormonal imbalance, diet and nutritional deficiencies, bacterial infection (including sexually transmitted diseases), and irritants such as chemicals or foreign objects.

Treatment: The most common cause of vaginitis is candida albicans. Herbal immune boosting support is important. A tincture made of 2 parts Echinacea angustifolia, 2 parts Goldenseal and 1 part Phytolacca, taken 30 to 60 drops (1 to 2 dropperfuls) every 2 to 4 hours helps relieve vaginits. Rinsing the vagina with apple cider vinegar (diluted to 50% with distilled water) can help relieve the itching almost immediately. Female herbs such as black cohosh, wild yam, angelica (dong quai) and chastetree berry. Take probiotics daily (Acidophilus or probiotic capsule or yogurt with an active culture). Garlic taken orally is one of the best natural antibiotics. Vaginal suppositories (called pessary). Use coconut butter to mix the following herbs into a wet pie dough consistency. - Equal parts Squaw vine herb, Slippery elm bark, Yellow dock root, Comfrey root, Marshmallow root, Chickweed herb, Goldenseal root, Mullein leaf (all powdered). Roll the herbs into pieces about an inch long about the diameter of your 5th finger (the pinky). Harden in a refrigerator and insert into the vagina over night. The pessary should be soft enough that it melts into the vagina. If it remains as a solid mass, you need to use less herb and more coconut butter. A sanitary napkin is advisable to use concurrently.

Prevention Tips:

1. Shower daily to keep vulva area clean.
2. Wipe from front to back after a bowel movement.
3. Keep vaginal area dry.
4. Wear cotton underwear. Avoid nylon pantyhose. Start using knee-highs.
5. Avoid using perfumed chemical douches or other perfumed or chemical products in the vaginal area.
6. Use condoms during sexual intercourse. Practice monogamy.

ENVIRONMENTAL INJURIES

CARBON-MONOXIDE POISONING - Smoke Inhalation

Definition/Diagnosis: Carbon monoxide is a colorless, odorless gas that kills without warning. A car engine left running in a closed garage can swiftly produce a lethal dose of carbon monoxide. The gas is also generated by wood, coal and charcoal fires, faulty oil burners, etc. In poorly ventilated rooms, the hazard of poisoning is present.

Symptoms of carbon-monoxide poisoning are: headache, dizziness, weakness, difficult breathing, possible vomiting, followed by collapse and unconsciousness. Skin, fingernail's and lips may be pink or cherry-red.

Treatment: Open all windows and doors and get the victim into fresh air immediately. Use cayenne pepper tincture 1 to 10 dropperful to revive the person and stimulate circulation. Use lobelia tincture 2 to 10 dropperfuls to aid in breathing. Begin artificial respiration promptly (see page 18) if they are not breathing or breathing irregularly, and begin CPR (see page 24) if breathing has stopped. Keep him lying quietly to prevent shock. Maintain normal body temperature. Call 911. Be sure to state the nature of the trouble and specify the need for oxygen because of carbon-monoxide poisoning.

Herbally begin using hawthorn berry syrup or hawthorn leaf tea. This increases the oxygen carrying capacity of the red blood cells. 3 to 6 cups of tea per day or 3 Tbs. of syrup per day.

CHILBLAINS

Definition/Diagnosis: This results when dry skin is exposed to temperatures from 60°F to freezing. The skin is red, swollen, frequently tender and itching. This is the mildest form of cold injury and no tissue loss results.

Treatment: Treat by preventing a repeat exposure and massage in Deep Heat ointment to warm and moisturize the skin. Drink warm herbal teas such as yarrow, ginger or peppermint.

DEHYDRATION

Definition/Diagnosis: Try this simple test. Pinch the back of you hand and let go quickly. Notice how quickly the skin recoils back to the normal position. When you are dehydrated the skin will fall back slower than normal. A dehydrated person will also have dried and/or cracked lips. Dehydration can cause a severe headache.

Treatment: See heat related conditions. Heat Cramps, page 151, Heat Exhaustion page 152, Diarrhea page 53, Headaches, page 115. Do not drink soda, sugared drinks, caffeinated drinks, or alcohol. These do not effectively rehydrate the body. Drink water with a pinch of natural sea salt or table salt in each glass or 1/8 teaspoon to every 12 to 16 ounces. It is important to replace the minerals (electrolytes) that are lost with perspiration and respiration.

ELECTRIC SHOCK

Every second of contact with the source of electricity lessens the victim's chance of survival. Break the victim's contact with the source of current in the quickest safe way possible. Indoors, disconnect the plug of the offending appliance, or pull the main switch at the fuse box. Outdoors, do not try to remove the victim from the wire yourself. Call the fire department and the local electric company and inform them of the emergency. Only qualified experts like line employees or fire-department crews trained for such situations can safely help the victim when the source of current is a power line.

Treatment: Don't touch any victim of electric shock until contact with the current has been broken. Then check to see if the victim is breathing and has a pulse. If necessary, administer artificial respiration (see page 18) or CPR (see page 24). Send for medical aid at once (Call 911). Check for burns or wounds at the current's entry and exit points.

If it is necessary to move the victim again, check to be sure the accident has not caused bone fractures or internal injuries. (See "Moving an Injured Person," page 37).

FISHHOOK REMOVAL

The first aid approach to an embedded fishhook is to tape it in place and not to try and remove it if there is any danger of causing damage to nearby or underlying body structure. Also do not try to remove it if the person is uncooperative. Cut the fish line off the hook. Cut off the remaining barbs of triple hooks.

If it looks like you will not be able to get medical help within 2 days, you must remove the fishhook yourself. This advice includes any impaled object, as the main risk is infection. Most fishhooks are pretty easy to remove anyway, so you may want to prevent the drive into town and the endless waiting in a doctors office or emergency room.

There are three basic methods of removing a fishhook.

Push through, snip off method - This technique is pretty straight forward. Keep in mind these points. 1) Pushing the hook through should not endanger underlying or adjacent structure. 2) Cleanse the skin at the anticipated second puncture site. 3) Punching a hook through the skin is a painful process. It hurts as much poking through the top of the skin as it does coming up and out from under the skin. Once you're committed, get it over in a hurry. 4) Skin is not easy to push through. It is very elastic and will pouch up over the barb as you try to push it through. Hold tissue down where the barb will come up. 5) Snip off the barb of the protruding point once it is through, then back the barb-less hook back out. 6) clean the two puncture wounds. See puncture wounds, page

198. If you do not have wire cutters, try to crush the barb flat enough to back the hook out.

The string jerk method - Do not use this method if the hook is embedded in the fingers or hand. The hands and fingers have many fine ligaments and tendons that could make this method difficult if not impossible. This technique works best in the back of the head, the shoulder, the back, chest, arms and legs. It can be virtually painless and causes minimal trauma.

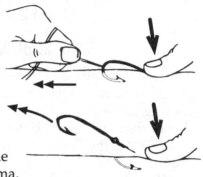

Loop some fishing line around the hook positioning the line so that it is flush with the skin. Push down on the eye portion of the hook. This will help to disengage the hook barb so that the quick pull will jerk the hook free with minimal trauma. Vigorously jerk the hook along the skin surface. Don't be surprised to finding the person asking when you are going to pull it out after you've completed.

The dissection method - Don't try this if you are at all able to get the person to help. This method would be necessary with embedded triple hooks, a hook near the eye or other situations where the previous two method cannot be used.

FROSTBITE

Definition/Diagnosis: Usually the most common freezing of the tissues exposed to the elements are the face, hands and feet. Watch for possible pain in the early stages. Just before frostbite occurs, the victim's skin may be flushed. As the condition develops the exposed part will become numb and turn white or grayish-yellow. In progressed stages blisters may appear on the skin. (Do not break any blisters).

The best thing for frostbite is prevention. Always bring extra clothing when hiking in cold weather and make sure hands and feet are kept dry and covered. (Use any type of insulation available, dry grass stuffed in gloves and boots works well in an emergency.)

Treatment: If frostbite is suspected:

1. Find shelter for the person, get them out of the elements. Take off any wet clothing. Wrap entire body in blankets, sleeping bags, coats, etc. to prevent hypothermia.

2. Do not rub frostbitten areas, as it can cause further damage. Also, re-freezing after re-warming can cause serious damage and should be avoided at all costs. A person can walk many miles on frozen feet, but as soon as the re-warming takes place, the person will be laid up and unable to walk until healing takes place. So make sure if you can't get to the hospital, that you can stay in one place until healed after re-warming of frostbitten areas.

3. In a remote area with no chance of getting to a hospital, warm up some water (104°-108° F, check by putting your hand in water and feel to where it is comfortably warm), add 1 Tbs. ginger powder and 2 Tbs. cayenne powder to 2 gallons. Soak frostbitten area in warm water solution for a least an hour or until frostbitten area becomes flushed. (If feet are involved, do not allow the person to walk).

4. During the re-warming, and afterwards, drink Nettle, Horsetail, Catnip, Mint tea or other warm liquids. Take 1 dropperful of Cayenne tincture under tongue.

Dry off frostbitten area very gently without rubbing. Separate toes or fingers by placing rolled gauze or clean cloth between them. Raise affected parts and keep from contact with bedclothes or other materials. Apply CTR Ointment after the pain is gone. Drink Nettle and Horsetail tea, 4-6 cups daily.

HEAT STRESS/HEAT CRAMPS

Definition/Diagnosis: High environmental temperature are frequently aggravated by the amount of work being done, the humidity, reflection of heat from rock, sand or other structures (even snow) and the lack of air movement. It takes a human about 10 days to become acclimated to the heat. Once heat stress adaptation take place, there will be a decrease in the loss of salt in the sweat. Once adapted the body will also sweat less. Salt can normally be replaced with food at mealtimes.

Salt depletion can result in nausea, twitching of muscle groups and at times severe cramping of abdominal muscles, legs, or elsewhere.

Treatment: Treatment consists of stretching the muscles involved (avoid aggressive massage), resting in a cool environment, and replacing salt losses. Generally 10-15 grams of salt in two quarts of water should do it. 5 grams is the weight of a nickel. So use 2-3 nickels worth. Drinking celery juice, carrot juice and watermelon is very effective.

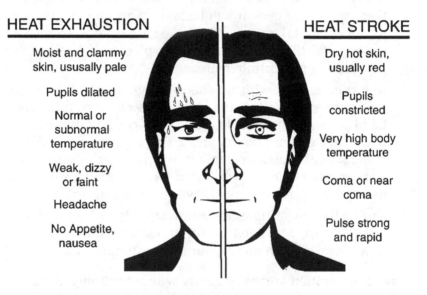

HEAT EXHAUSTION

Moist and clammy skin, ususally pale

Pupils dilated

Normal or subnormal temperature

Weak, dizzy or faint

Headache

No Appetite, nausea

HEAT STROKE

Dry hot skin, usually red

Pupils constricted

Very high body temperature

Coma or near coma

Pulse strong and rapid

HEAT EXHAUSTION

Definition/Diagnosis: Less serious than heat stroke, but unless treated can escalate to the life threatening heat stroke. Symptoms include headache, extreme fatigue, dizziness, cold clammy and pale skin, sometimes fainting - but normal or only slightly elevated temperature. Heat exhaustion can be treated by rest in a shaded area or air-conditioned room.

Treatment: Have the person lie down with legs and feet raised 8 to 12 inches higher than the level of his head. Place cold towels on his head, but avoid chilling. Give sips of cool, diluted salt water (1/2 tsp. added to each cup). Drink at least 4 ounces every 15 minutes. Orange juice or celery juice is also helpful. Don't give fluids if the victim becomes nauseated, until nausea subsides.

HEAT - PRICKLY HEAT

Definition/Diagnosis: This is a heat rash caused by the entrapment of sweat in glands in the skin. This can result in irritation and frequently severe itching.

Treatment: Include cooling and drying the involved area and avoiding conditions that may induce sweating for awhile. Keep well hydrated (Drink 10-12 cups per day). Several hours of cool, dry environment daily is the only reliable treatment for prickly heat. Use Herbal Pain formula for itching. The sensation of itching follows pain nerve fibers and responds well to herbs that reduce pain.

HEAT STROKE

Definition/Diagnosis: The body can suffer a number of reactions when exposed to excessive heat. The elderly, chronic invalids, very young, alcoholics, and people who are over weight are the most likely to suffer from heat stroke. Heatstroke may happen with strenuous activity when there is high temperatures. Always drink plenty of liquids while doing strenuous activities in hot weather.

Heat stroke (body temperature of 105°-106° F) is a very serious medical emergency. The victim of heat stroke is weak, irritable, dazed, nauseated. Sweating stops; skin becomes hot, red and dry. The victim may lose consciousness. Heat stroke is life threatening.

Treatment: Body temperature must be lowered immediately. Immerse patient in cold-water bath, stream or lake with clothing removed. Or use a sponge or cloth soaked in cold water to cool the skin. If outdoors, place the victim in a shaded place and cool him off as quickly as possible. Use a garden hose - running water is an ideal cooling method. If no hose is available, pour cool water over the victim - buckets of cool water. If the person is conscious, give cool drinks but no stimulants such as drinks containing alcohol or caffeine. Check temperature every 5-10 minutes until it drops to 100°-102° F. (If no thermometer, until person feels normal to touch. Do not overchill).

During and after the cooling down process, have the person lie or sit in a shaded area, out of the sun. If temperature begins to rise again, repeat the cooling process. If the person gets chilled, cover with a blanket.

Symptoms of heat stroke are very high body temperature (104° - 106° F), absence of sweating, skin is hot, red and dry. Person may be in a stupor or perhaps unconscious.

CAUTION: Do not give the person any stimulants (alcohol, coffee, tea, etc.)

After the body temperature is lowered (102° F) and the person is no longer in a stupor, drink 1-2 cups of celery juice. If this is not available, drink 4-8 cups of cool water with 1/2 tsp. salt added to each cup.

Cooling is the first step, but quickly call an ambulance. Get the victim of heat stroke to a hospital emergency room as soon as possible.

HYPOTHERMIA

Definition/Diagnosis: The number one concept in the woods for survival is to stay calm, dry and warm. With most wilderness medical problems, prevention is always more important than treatment. If you do become cold, wet or exhausted, find or make a shelter where you are out of the harsh elements.

Two of the greatest dangers of hypothermia are physical exhaustion and wet clothing. People who are the most likely to succumb to hypothermia are those of a thin body type (usually male) who lack sufficient body fat to help insulate against the cold.

Symptoms of hypothermia are fatigue, shivering, goose bumps, hallucinations, disorientation, drowsiness, slurred speech, and low body temperature (91°-98° F). If any of these symptoms occur, find shelter immediately out of the elements, and begin treatment for hypothermia. With hypothermia, death can occur in a surprisingly short time (a few hours), even when the temperatures are not freezing, but it is windy and the person is wet, malnourished, or not clothed properly. Watch the breathing and apply artificial respiration if necessary. Hypothermia is common when there are head injuries, blood loss, a fracture and the person is immobilized in cold weather, and in shock.

Treatment: for Mild Hypothermia: (body temp. 95° F or higher) make sure the person is in dry clothing, adding more clothes, blankets, or sleeping bags to keep warm. Administer 1 dropperful of Cayenne tincture and Nettles Tincture and give warm teas made from ginger, Nettles and yarrow sweetened with honey. (Hot soup or drinks can be used if herbs are not available). Keep person out of wind and elements in a proper shelter. Apply Deep Heat ointment or oil to chest, neck, back, feet and hands. (avoid eyes or sensitive areas).

Treatment for Moderate Hypothermia: (body temp. 90°-94° F). Treat the same as mild hypothermia except additional heat needs to be provided as fast as possible to the person's body without burning them. One of the best ways is to get one or two persons that are warm into a sleeping bag (like a cocoon) with the person, skin to skin contact. This will bring up the persons body core temperature quickly and safely. Hot water bottles, warm baths, warm stones, or any other safe heat source can also be used.

If you don't have a thermometer and can't tell the severity of the hypothermia, treat as if moderate to severe. (Don't give teas if unconscious).

When shivering stops (when the body temperature is rising), it is a good sign. But if it stops when the body temperature is falling, it is a bad sign. Shivering is the body's way of producing heat.

Symptoms of Severe Hypothermia: Body temperature is 80°-90° F, muscles are rigid, gross incoordination occurs; mental activity dulls; unresponsiveness (coma), pulse and respiration slows down. Body temperature below 80° F is life threatening, with irregularities of the heart. Few persons survive body temperatures below 75° F.

The important thing to remember in all cases of hypothermia is that the body's central core (the torso) is warmed first before warming the extremities. It is dangerous to warm the arms and legs before the central part of the body is heated! With severe hypothermia use your judgment on how much cayenne or shepherd's purse tincture to give. Be willing to do whatever it takes to get the body core temperature up and the circulation moving.

In severe cases of hypothermia, do not treat the victim if hospitalization is available. There are sophisticated treatments to warm these potentially lethal cases that hospitals are equipped for.

Cayenne Tincture - 1 dropperful under the tongue. In all cases of hypothermia, the body core temperature must be warmed as quickly and safely as possible (Direct body contact, warm baths, warm drinks, etc.) Do not warm extremities before the body core is warmed. Keep victim in adequate shelter, away from wind and elements. Make sure they are dry and comfortable.

LIGHTNING

Definition/Diagnosis: Lightning kills more people every year in the United States than all other natural disasters combined. Carrying or wearing metal objects, such as umbrella, back pack or even a hairpin, increases the chances of being hit.

To calculate the approximate distance in miles from a flash of lightning, count in seconds (one one thousand, two one thousand, etc.) from when you see the flash to when you hear the thunder, then divide by five. In other words, five seconds per mile from flash to thunder.

Other than being fried and killed instantly, cardiopulmonary arrest is the most significant lightning injury. People who are screaming from fright or burns after lightning are demonstrating that they are okay and out of immediate danger. Their wounds can be tended to later. Those who appear dead must have immediate attention. Burns from lightning itself are generally not severe. After the heart and breathing consequences of a lightning strike, neurological defects are the secondary concern. 72% of victims lose consciousness and 75% will have a cardiac arrest. Most will have amnesia and confusion and a short term memory loss that may last two to five days after the injury.

Lightning can cause injury by four mechanisms:

1. Direct Hit - lightning directly strikes a person in the open. It usually doesn't enter the body, but instead is conducted over the skin surface called a "flashover". The greatest damage is usually a burn to the skin underneath metal objects such as zippers, jewelry or belt buckles. The current can also penetrate deeper parts of the body through the eyes, ears, and mouth causing disruption to the brain,

lungs or heart. The instant vaporization of any moisture on the person's skin can blast apart the clothing and shoes.

2. Splash - When a bolt first hits an object such as a tree or another person, it can jump to another person who may have even found shelter.

3. Step Voltage - when lightning hits the ground or a nearby object the current can spread like a ripples in a pond. Several people can be hurt this way by a single bolt of lightning.

4. Blunt Trauma - The explosive force of the pressure waves created by lightning, can cause blunt trauma, like ruptured ear drums, or spleen or liver injuries.

Treatment: Lightning victims are not "charged" and pose no threats to any rescuer. Treat for respiratory or heart failure with CPR and/or rescue breathing. Treat for burns as necessary. Stabilize and splint any fractures. Treat for spinal injury or injury due to blunt trauma as necessary. Begin using Nerve Repair Formula 4 dropperfuls 6 times daily. Monitor vital signs for the next 24 to 48 hours.

POISONING (By Mouth)

First, identify the poison if possible. Call your poison control center or hospital emergency room immediately. Tell what the suspected poison is and get specific instructions.

IN GENERAL: Don't induce vomiting if the victim has swallowed a strong corrosive poison such as carbolic acid, toilet bowl cleaner, lye, drain cleaner, or ammonia. Also do not induce vomiting if the victim is asleep or is having a seizure. Give plenty of fresh water or milk to drink. If it is not a strong corrosive poison or petroleum product, induce vomiting by giving them 1-3 teaspoons of Lobelia Tincture, or by gagging with finger in the back of their throat. Use Colon Detox powder mixed in water to neutralize the poison (1-2 teaspoons in 1 cup of water). Then use Immune Boost Formula 1-2 dropperfuls every hour. Keep the person calm and warm, sitting up in a comfortable position. If unconscious or convulsing, do not administer anything by mouth, but seek medical attention immediately.

Some other suggestions:

Food Poisoning: Use Burdock root tea to neutralize and eliminate poisons. Horehound tea is said to be an excellent antidote for all types of seafood poisoning, especially poisoning from crab or lobster. Horehound is used for poisoning from E. coli and salmonella as well.

Drug Overdoes and Addiction: The key here is to neutralize and detoxify. A tea made of one part each comfrey, mullein, and spearmint with half parts rosehips and orange peel then a pinch of goldenseal added just before drinking. This will not only clean out the opiates from the body but reduce the desire for more. Using colon detox as described above is also very effective in drawing the toxins out of the system. Use a green drink such as SuperNutrition 3 times daily. To treat the effects of withdrawal make a tea consisting of equal parts valerian, chamomile and catnip (or peppermint or spearmint).

Household Cleaning Agents (lye, toilet bowl cleaner, etc.): Dilute, dilute, dilute. Drink as much milk or water as possible. Use colon detox to absorb poisons. Olive oil, fenugreek seed and slippery elm teas will help to ease the pain.

Poisonous Plants: Use colon detox to absorb toxins. Also a strong tea that his high in tannins such as white oak bark is useful. Protect the liver from mushroom poisoning with milk thistle seed. Make a strong tea. Drink 1 gallon of this tea in 24 hours. It will save your liver and your life.

Heavy Metals: Burdock root tea, Oregon grape root tea, Milk thistle tea or tincture, Goldenseal, even some blue cheeses like gorgonzola are good for lead poisoning. For lead poisoning look for a bluish line or tint in the gums above the teeth. Garlic and onions are good for lead and cadmium poisoning especially with cases of slow accumulation. Foods such as milk and eggs will inactivate mercury located within the body.

Insecticides (DDT, and related herbicides): Kelp and other herbs high in sodium should be taken after the initial crisis is over. Use the colon detox for 5-7 days as described on page 158, or follow the detox program on page 257.

For arsenic poisoning, use large amounts of burdock root tea, strong black coffee, or plain sagebrush tea. All are excellent remedies.

RADIATION POISONING or SICKNESS

Definition/Diagnosis: Radiation sickness is caused by exposure to radioactive substances. Radiation can kill, damage or cause cells to mutate becoming cancerous.

Treatment: The seaweed kelp can absorb a lot of radiation from within the body. Other seaweed's such as Dulse, Irish moss, and Iceland moss work similarly. Clay (Bentonite) and apple pectin also absorbs radioactive isotopes within the body. Colon Detox powder used 5 - 6 times daily for 5-7 days.(1 tsp. per 12 oz. water - the taste is not as bad as the texture, just slam it down fast before it begins to gel up). St. Johnswort, garlic, slippery elm and fenugreek, and aloe vera are all known to reduce the damaging effects of radiation.

Drink Miso soup 4-6 cups daily. American Ginseng Tincture 15-20 drops 3 times daily.

Bathe in 2 pounds of Epsom's Salt water for 1 hour, then 2 pounds of soda water for 1 hour. Eat foods naturally high in Iodine or Selenium. Eat broccoli, cauliflower, Brussels sprouts, cabbage. Eliminate all dairy products except yogurt.

SNOW BLINDNESS

Definition/Diagnosis: This is a severely painful condition caused by ultraviolet B rays of the sun which are reflected by the snow (85% reflection), water (10-100%), and sand (17%). Thin cloud layers allow this wavelength of light to filter through without the infrared (heat) rays of the sun coming through. Because of this it can be a cool and overcast day with bright snow and cause a sunburned eye or snow blindness. You don't need to be in the snow to suffer from snow blindness.

Of course prevention is the key. Always wear properly approved (ANSI) sunglasses which will block 99.8% of the UV B wavelength light. Even a backup pair can be a good idea. If glasses are lost or unavailable slit glasses can be made from wood, a bandanna or many materials available.

Snow blindness is a self-limited affliction. However, not only is the loss of vision a problem, but so is the terrible pain. It is described as hot pokers in the eyes.

Treatment: Herbal eyewash can be soothing as also CTR oil or ointment put into the eyes. Usually both eyes are equally afflicted, if not patch just the one eye. However, generally both eyes should be patched and the patient should rest anywhere from 1 to 5 days using ointment and wash 3-5 times daily.

SUNBURN

If the skin is reddened but not blistered, apply cold, wet compresses to the sunburned area to relieve pain or submerge in cold water. Do not use butter or margarine, these may irritate or introduce infection. Apply fresh Aloe Vera gel to the area. This is both soothing and healing. If the skin is blistered or extensively burned cover it with a wet cloth of water. Severe or extensive sunburn may require medical assistance particularly if infection occurs. Apply Aloe Vera gel or CTR Ointment over the burn every 4-6 hours. For more severe sunburns we recommend CTR Ointment or Dr. Christopher's Burn Formula (equal parts honey, wheat germ oil and comfrey leaf, blended into a paste).

Chapter 11

INFECTIOUS DISEASES

Microorganisms are everywhere: in the soil, water and air. Everyday we eat, drink and breathe them. Yet it is rare that these organisms invade, multiply and produce infections in humans. When we do get an infection often they are so mild, we don't even have symptoms. Occasionally, a microorganism (bacteria, virus, parasites, etc.) will gain a foothold in our bodies causing a infection. This triggers an immune response to fight and eliminate the infection. The key to overcoming an infection is to boost the immune system so that the body will eliminate the invading organism and kill or destroy the organism directly. The primary tool in the medical arsenal is antibiotics. The overuse and abuse of antibiotics have resulted in virulent bacteria that are resistant to antibiotics and are even more difficult to fight naturally.

Of the following conditions that are discussed, many are fatal if untreated. If a potentially fatal infectious illness occurs, treat aggressively with herbal protocols, such as Anti-Plague Syrup, The Cold Sheet Treatment, and the Incurables Checklist. Fresh garlic taken in quantities from 6 to 50 cloves daily is powerful and effective in killing "germs". Echinacea will boost the immune system. You will notice that the same treatment is recommended for many of these diseases. The principle to learn here is that our objective is build and strengthen the body so that the body will effectively fight the disease and heal itself, rather than trying to attack the organism with a drug we hope will be effective. Please note that many of these conditions are potentially life threatening and medical assistance can offer the quickest and safest solution.

BABESIOSIS (Tick Bite)

Definition/Diagnosis: This is a malaria-like illness caused by a protozoan parasite that invades the red blood cells. Symptoms gradually begin one week after a tick bite with fatigue and loss of appetite giving way in several days to fever, drenching sweats, muscle ache and headache. The illness ranges from mild to severe, with death occurring in about 10% of patients.

Treatment: Treat with immune boosting herbs taken hourly, and the Cold Sheet Treatment. Follow Incurables checklist.

BLASTOMYCOSIS (Fungus)

Definition/Diagnosis: This infectious disease is caused by a fungus. Outbreaks usually occur in the southeastern United States, or various parts of Africa. Onset of the illness is slowly progressive, usually starting with a cough and developing into a pneumonia with fevers, shortness of breath, chest pain, and drenching sweats. Infected blood carries the fungus to the skin and other tissues. Skin lesions enlarge with a collapsed center, purplish-red border and frequent ulcerations. In most untreated patients the disease is slowly progressive and fatal.

Treatment: Immune boosting herbs, Cold Sheet Treatment and Incurables protocol.

CHOLERA (Bacteria)

Definition/Diagnosis: This acute intestinal infection is caused by a bacterium (Vibrio cholerae) which produces profuse, cramping diarrhea, muscular cramps and suppression of urine. Symptoms develop rapidly and can become dangerous in 6 to 12 hours. Children may be restless and go into a stupor and have seizures. Death usually comes from dehydration. Drinking contaminated water cause the disease to spread. This infection occurs world wide. Vaccination is ineffective. The strain of cholera raging in most of the world is resistant to antibiotics.

Treatment: Oral re-hydration is vital. See diarrhea, page 53. Boost immune system with anti-plague syrup and immune enhancing herbs. Use colon detox to absorb toxins and slow the bowel. Rice water will check the diarrhea as will peach leaves, raspberry leaves and sunflower leaves. A warm cat-nip enema is very soothing and will calm the cramping spasms within the bowel. Slippery Elm made into a gruel should also be eaten. Two tablespoons slippery elm to 1/2 cup of water.

COCCIDIOIDOMYCOSIS (Fungus)

Definition/Diagnosis: This fungal infection is found in the San Joaquin Valley in California as well as in the southwestern United States. The disease spreads by inhaling the fungal spore in dust. Onset of the disease can be weeks, months, or even years after the original infection (particularly in an immunodepressed person). The primary symptoms are an upper respiratory infection such as bronchitis or pneumonia.

Treatment: Treat as you would an upper respiratory infection, see page 95, as well as with immune enhancing herbs or remedies. Cold Sheet Treatment and Incurables Checklist are also appropriate.

COLDS/FLU (Virus)

Definition/Diagnosis: While not a strict emergency, there are conditions that can begin like or mimic a cold or the flu so swift treatment can be very appropriate. The potentially deadly biologic agent "anthrax" during the first day or so can look like the flu. Normally a cold and the flu are nature's way to cleanse the body. Support this cleansing process, rather than take drugs to suppress the symptoms (which, by the way, are a necessary part of cleaning the body).

Treatment: Stop eating solid foods. Drink one gallon of Red Raspberry leaf tea in a 24 hour period. Take 1-2 dropperfuls of Immune Boost Tincture every waking hour or 1 Tablespoon of Anti-Plague Formula every waking hour. Take Colon Cleanse (page 222) if necessary. Absolutely no sweets, this includes fruit juices. Administration of the Cold Sheet Treatment (see page 248) or even a modified version of it will rapidly speed your recovery. See Boosting Your Immune System page 246.

COLORADO TICK FEVER (Tick)

Definition/Diagnosis: This viral disease is spread by ticks and is 20 times more common than Rocky Mountain Spotted Fever in Colorado. In can be found in all states of the Western Rockies and Western Canada. It is most frequent in April-May at low altitude and June-July at high altitudes. Remove tick or identify the site of the bite.

Onset is abrupt, with chills, fever of 100.4° F to 104° F, muscle ache, headache, eye pain, and eye sensitivity to light. The patient feels weak and nauseated, but vomiting is unusual. During the first 2 days, up to 12% of the victims develop a rash. In half the cases the fever disappears after 2 to 3 days and the patient feels well for 2 days. Then a second bout of illness starts which lasts intensely for 2 to 4 days. The second phase subsides with the patient feeling weak for 1 to 2 additional weeks. The same tick spreads Rocky Mountain Spotted Fever which requires more aggressive treatment.

Treatment: Traditionally treated with bed rest, fluids to prevent dehydration and pain medication for fever and aches. Treat with immune boosting herbs, cold sheet treatment and incurables checklist.

CRYPTOSPORIDIOSIS - CRYPTO (Parasite)

Definition/Diagnosis: This microscopic parasite (similar to Giardia) lives in the feces of infected humans and animals. It is found in nearly all surface waters that have been tested nationwide. Crypto is a resilient parasite that is not killed by chlorine or iodine at concentrations normally used to disinfect drinking water. Very fine filter or boiling water will kill this bug. Symptoms include abdominal cramping, low-grade fever, nausea, vomiting and diarrhea (which can lead to dehydration). Illness begins 2 to 7 days after drinking infected water and can last two to three weeks before it resolves on its own. It can be fatal to the immunodepressed.

Treatment: Treat as you would parasites, see page 172. Treat dehydration as necessary.

DENGUE - Breakbone Fever, Dandy fever (Mosquito)

Definition/Diagnosis: This viral infection is spread by mosquito bites. Dengue is endemic (constantly present) in the tropics and subtropics. Fever begins 3 to 15 days (usually 5 to 8 days) after exposure. Fever is accompanied by chills, headache, low back ache, pain behind the eyes with movement of the eyes, extreme aching in the legs and joints. The eyes are red and a flushing or pale pink rash can occur on the face. There is a relatively slow pulse rate for the high body temperature. The pulse rate typically will increase as the body temperature rises. The fever last 48 to 96 hours, followed by a 24 hour period of no fever and a sense of well being. Then a second rapid fever occurs (typically not as high as the first fever). A bright rash spreads from the arms/legs to the trunk, but generally not the face. Palms and soles may be bright red and swollen. There is a severe headache and other body aches as well. The fever, rash, and headache constitute the "dengue triad" which distinguish this disease from others. The illness lasts for weeks, but has no mortality rate (it won't kill you). However, a condition called Dengue Hemorrhagic Fever Shock Syndrome is lethal and occurs in patients younger than 10. Primarily in infants under one year of age. Dengue can be confused with Colorado tick fever, typhus, yellow fever or other hemmorrhagic fevers.

Treatment: Treat with bedrest and immune supporting herbs (echinacea, goldenseal, cat's claw, and formulae such as antiplague and immune boost). Cold Sheet Treatment is not necessary, but will speed the recovery.

DYSENTERY (Protozoa)

Definition/Diagnosis: This infection of the colon is characterized by diarrhea and the passage of blood, pus and mucus in the stools, which are highly infectious. Dysentery may be caused by protozoans or bacteria that are spread chiefly in water or food. The symptoms include griping pains in the intestines, constant strain to evacuate the bowels, and intense diarrhea. Often there will be fever, sleeplessness, lack of appetite, swollen abdomen, rapid breathing, slow pulse and hot urine.

Treatment: Treat as you would for diarrhea and parasites. In addition, if there is bleeding from the bowel, mullein leaf heated in milk will speed healing. A warm high enema of white oak bark or bayberry bark will calm the diarrhea. Fomentation of castor oil with lobelia tincture will ease the pain. Slippery elm gruel and oatmeal water should be taken in.

ENCEPHALITIS (Mosquito)

Definition/Diagnosis: There are two groups or classifications of encephalitis; Group A and Group B Arbovirus. The person is infected from the bite of an infected mosquito. Symptoms include high fever (104° F), a generalized headache, stiff neck, vomiting and at times diarrhea. Encephalitis can be fatal. Be very careful of mosquito exposure if an outbreak occurs.

Treatment: Cool the patient with water. Boost the immune system. Perform the Cold Sheet Treatment.

FEVER - CHILLS

Definition/Diagnosis: Fever is not a disease, but an elevation in body temperature. However it may indicate the presence of disease. Frequently "fevers of unknown origin" are associated with Salmonella or Shigella infections. As a fever increases above normal, the white blood cell activity or immune response increases. Therefore, supporting a fever during an infectious illness rather than trying to eliminate it is important. The most important thing to remember during a fever is to keep the person well hydrated. As long as the person is drinking enough fluids (water, herb teas, etc.), the fever should not cause any harm or damage. Constipation and congestion will keep a fever up. As long as a fever does not get too high (above 103° F, some say 104° F) let it run its course. See a health care professional if you observe the following;

Treatment: Review Boosting your Immune System page 246. Some procedures that are useful during fever may be:

1. Avoid Solid foods. Drink plenty of fluid. At least 1 cup per hour.
2. Perform the Cold Sheet Treatment and use immune building herbal formula such as Immune Boost Formula, Anti-Plague Formula
3. Force plenty of fluids (herbal tea).
4. Soak in a hot Ginger bath (1/2 cup powdered ginger in tub).
5. Slippery Elm tea is good for settling your stomach in all cases of fever.

6. Cool water enemas can help remove poisons from the system.

7. Lobelia Tincture 1-3 Tbs. Until it produces vomiting if necessary (see lobelia purge, page 95).

8. Yarrow, Elderflower, or Peppermint Tincture: 10-15 drops 3 times a day are good diaphoretics (promotes sweating).

GIARDIASIS (Parasite)

Definition/Diagnosis: This is an intestinal infection caused by a single cell parasite. It is becoming more and more prevalent throughout the world. It is spread through contamination of fecal material into water that is ingested. About two weeks after ingestion the Giardia cysts hatch producing either a gradual or abrupt onset of persistent watery diarrhea which is sometimes described as explosive. Abdominal pain, bloating, nausea, and weight loss from malabsorption may occur. Symptoms resolve in one to two weeks, but can persist in a chronic state for several months.

Treatment: Treat as you would a parasitic infection (see parasites/worms, page 172).

GLANDS (Swollen Lymph Nodes)

Definition/Diagnosis: Swollen glands or fluid filled cysts can be effectively reduced and either reabsorbed by the body or brought to a head and expelled by the body.

Treatment: Mullein 3 parts & Lobelia 1 part as an oil. Massage into swollen gland. Mullein and lobelia taken internally is also recommended in either tea, tincture, capsule or even the oil. Deep Heat oil massaged into area then apply CTR Ointment.

HANTAVIRUS (Dust)

Definition/Diagnosis: This virus is caught by inhaling the dust of contaminated feces from an infected deer mouse. The onset of the illness begins with a period of fever, muscle ache and a cough followed by an abrupt onset of acute respiratory distress. The mortality rate has been up to 60%. Medicine has no specific treatment available other than avoid breathing the dust that is contaminated.

Treatment: Of course prevention is always recommended, however to insure that you are in the 40% that will survive this, it is important to boost your immune system, cleanse the elimination channels (colon, liver, kidney's, skin and lungs).

Perform the Cold Sheet Treatment, hourly anti-plague syrup and/or immune boost. Lobelia tincture is the herb of choice for acute respiratory distress.

HEPATITIS A - Infectious Hepatitis (Food/Water)

Definition/Diagnosis: Hepatitis is an inflammation of the liver. The liver becomes tender and enlarged. Palpate under the lower border of the right ribs. If you can feel the liver easily and it is tender, it is probably enlarged and inflamed.

This viral infection of the liver affects people worldwide. It is transmitted by ingestion of infected feces, either through water supplies contaminated by human feces, food handled by a person with poor hygiene, or contaminated food such as raw shellfish grown in impure water. Contaminated Milk and infected blood can also spread this disease.

The period from the time of exposure to the appearance of symptoms takes 15 to 50 days. The disease can range from minor flu-like symptoms to a fatal liver disease. Most cases self resolve within 6 to 12 weeks. Symptoms start abruptly with fever, lethargy, and nausea. Occasionally a rash will develop. A characteristic loss of taste for cigarettes is frequent. Of course, this is presuming you have a taste for cigarettes. In 3 to 10 days the urine turns dark, followed by jaundice or yellowing of the whites of the eyes and skin. The stool may turn a light color. There is frequently itching and joint pain. The jaundice peaks within one or two weeks and fades during the two to four week recovery phase. The 'Hepatitis A" patient stops shedding the virus as a carrier in the stool prior to the jaundice developing and is no longer contagious by the time the diagnosis is made. Personal hygiene is essential to prevent the spread of this disease.

Treatment: Medically no specific treatment is required. After a few days to 2 weeks the appetite generally returns and bed confinement is no longer required even though the jaundice still remains. The best gauge to recovery is the patients improving energy level. Diet should be low fat (see Health

Promoting Diet, page 243). Milk thistle seed should be taken abundantly (3 to 4 dropperfuls of tincture taken 4 to 5 times daily). This herb is specific for the liver, is completely safe and non toxic. Immune supporting herbs and formulae should be taken. SuperNutrition taken as directed 2 to 3 times daily is recommended. The Cold Sheet Treatment is also of benefit. Apply warm castor oil packs over the liver area. Keep warm with a hot water bottle. Keep the pack in place for 1/2 to two hours, as needed for pain relief.

HEPATITIS B - Serum Hepatitis (Sex/Blood)

Definition/Diagnosis: This viral liver disease is also world-wide in its distribution. Transmission is primarily through sexual contact, infected blood, use of needles, syringes, or even sharing contaminated razor blades. Dental procedures, acupuncture, ear piercing and tattooing with contaminated equipment will also spread the disease.

Incubation time from the exposure is longer than hepatitis A, usually 30 to 180 days. The symptoms are similar, but the onset is less abrupt and the incidence of fever is lower. There is a greater chance of developing chronic hepatitis (5-10% of cases). Mortality is higher, especially in the elderly or the immunosuppressed.

Treatment: Treat as you would hepatitis A.

HEPATITIS C - Non-A, Non-B (Sex/Blood)

Definition/Diagnosis: This form of hepatitis is similar to hepatitis B. It is transmitted the same ways as hepatitis B. Incubation is from two weeks to 25 weeks with an average of 7 weeks. Medicine has no specific treatment.

Treatment: Treat as you would hepatitis A.

LICE

Cover head for 2-3 hours with mayonnaise. Cover head with a shower cap to hold all of the goopy mayonnaise on. This will suffocate the lice. Comb hair with a fine comb to remove nits. Lice cannot live for more than 24 hours without human contact. Quarantine bedrooms where lice may be for 24 hours. Have everyone sleep in the living room to allow lice to die off in the other rooms. Many will opt to use over-the-counter shampoo and pesticides to kill the lice. These are becoming increasingly less effective as the population of lice are adapting to these poisons. If you choose to use a medicated shampoo, be sure and support and protect the liver by taking Milk Thistle seed and boost the immune system with Echinacea. Check everyone's head for nits for several days. Thyme essential oil rubbed through the hair kills lice and will prevent infection.

LYME DISEASE (Tick)

Definition/Diagnosis: This disease is transmitted by the bite of a tick and is found throughout the world. The disease goes through several phases. In Stage One, after an incubation of 3 days to a month, the person develops a circular lesion in the area of the bite. It has a clear to pink center, raised borders, is painless and ranges from 1 to 23 inches in diameter. There are usually several of these lesions. The person feels lethargic, has headaches, muscle and joint pain and enlarged lymph nodes. In Stage Two, 10-15% of people can develop meningitis, and less than 10% heart problems. Symptoms may last for months, but are generally self limiting (meaning it gets better on its own). About 60% experience Stage Three, which is the development of arthritis. Often the knee is involved. The swelling can be profound. Stage Three can begin suddenly after several weeks to 2 years after the initial rash. Bell's Palsy (one sided facial paralysis) is one possible manifestation of Lyme disease. The involved side is expressionless with the person being unable to move the muscles of the forehead, around the eye, or the face. While there are other causes to Bell's Palsy, if a patient presents you with this, you should not rule out Lyme disease.

Treatment: Treat as you would any infectious disease, with Immune boosting herbs, the cold sheet treatment and the incurable checklist. BioSET treatments can be effective.

MALARIA (Mosquito)

Definition/Diagnosis: Human malaria is caused by one of four protozoa (Plasmodium flaciparum, P. vivax, P. ovale, and P. malariae) transmitted from the bite of an infected female mosquito. It can also be spread by blood transfusion. This disease is potentially lethal, particularly the P.

flaciparum. There are many drugs that are used prophylactically, but are becoming largely ineffective as the protozoa develop resistance to these. Symptoms usually begin 10 to 35 days after a mosquito infects the parasite into the person. Often the first symptoms are a mild fever that comes and goes, headache, muscle ache, chills, and a general feeling of malaise (you just feel ill). Sometimes the symptoms begin with shaking chills followed by fever. These symptoms are often mistaken for the flu. Falciparum malaria can effect the brain causing a high fever 104° F, severe headache, drowsiness, delirium and confusion. This is the type of malaria that can be fatal.

Treatment: Boost the immune system (anti-plague syrup, immune boost) and build the blood (SuperNutrition, chlorophyll, "green drinks"). Cold Sheet Treatment and Incurable checklist is appropriate.

MENINGITIS - Meningococcal Meningitis
(bacterial, airborne)

Definition/Diagnosis: This acute bacterial infection causes inflammation in the linings of the brain and central nervous system. Many cases are without symptoms or consist of a mild upper respiratory illness. Severe cases begin with a sudden fever, sore throat, chills, headache, stiff neck, nausea, and vomiting. Flexing the head forward will greatly aggravate the headache and should alert you to this condition. Within 24 to 48 hours the person becomes drowsy, mentally confused, followed by convulsions, coma, and death. The disease is spread by contact with the nasal secretions of the infected person, usually through coughing and sneezing.

Treatment: This is a condition that should receive emergency medical treatment and responds well to high doses of antibiotics if treated early enough. If medical help is not available, treat very aggressively with Anti-Plague Syrup (1 Tbs. hourly), Cold Sheet Treatment, and the Incurables Checklist.

MONONUCLEOSIS - Infectious mononucleosis
(bacterial/Oral)

Definition/Diagnosis: This disease of young adults (from teens through 30 years of age), generally presents as a terrible sore throat, swollen lymph nodes (normally at the back of the neck and not as tender as with Strep infection), and a profound tired feeling. It is self-limited with total recovery expected from two weeks to six months. Spleen enlargement is common. The most serious aspect of this disease is the possibility of the spleen rupturing, but this is rare. Avoid palpating the spleen (shoving on the left upper quadrant of the abdomen), let the person rest until the illness and feeling of lethargy has passed. The first five days are typically the worst, with fever and excruciating sore throat being the major complaint. A mild form of hepatitis frequently occurs with mononucleosis that causes nausea and loss of appetite. Treat as you would mono. If severe ear pain begins use the herbal ear drops and moist heat over the ear. Strep throat can also be a concern, however the treatment described below is also very effective for Strep throat as well as mononucleosis.

Treatment: With aggressive juicing and use of nutritional and immune supporting herbs recovery from mono can be greatly accelerated. Drink 2 - 4 quarts of carrot juice daily. SuperNutrition 3 times daily. Immune Boost and/or Anti-Plague formula every waking hour. The more you do the speedier the recovery. Rest and do not encourage the person to over exert themselves. Lobelia tincture taken every 1/2 to 1 hour (3 to 10 drops depending on your size) is said to prevent mononucleosis.

PARASITES

Definition/Diagnosis: Technically any organism that lives off of another can be defined as a parasite. Parasites can range from single-cell organisms called protozoa to insects (arthropods) to worms. Illness can result when these disease-promoting parasites contaminate our food and water supply. Parasites can also infest the skin, as with scabies and lice, or can enter the bloodstream through insect bites as with malaria or yellow fever. Parasites deplete the body of essential nutrients and tax and overwhelm the body's immune system. Conditions such as Crohn's disease, ulcerative colitis, arthritis, chronic fatigue syndrome (CFS), Fibromyalgia, irritable bowel syndrome and many cases of diarrhea are all being links to parasites. Dr. Hulda Clark in her book *The Cure for All Disease* teaches that there are only two causes to health problems; Parasites and Pollution. While this view may be rather simplistic, there is a lot of truth to what she has to say. Parasites are a common causes of diarrhea and general intestinal upset.

Common symptoms of a parasitic infection can include, explosive or watery diarrhea, intermittent diarrhea and constipation, indigestion, rashes, hives, gas, fatigue, and allergic reactions to food. If left untreated arthritis symptoms may emerge. Mucous in stools, weight loss, constipation, nausea, vomiting, malabsorbtion, malnutrition, night sweats and fever may also occur. The toxicity from parasites can cause blackouts, muscular and skeletal pain, wide swings in blood sugar levels and menstrual irregularities.

Prevention: There are many things you can do to avoid parasites;

- Don't eat raw or undercooked beef - it can be loaded with tapeworms or other parasites.
- Don't eat raw fish (sushi or sashimi) - you are almost certain to get worms.
- Wash your hands thoroughly after handling any raw meats.
- Use a separate cutting board for meat and vegetables to avoid any cross contamination.
- Wash utensils after cutting meat.
- Wash fruit and vegetables thoroughly
- Don't sleep near your pets - they harbor many worms and other parasites.
- Deworm your pets regularly (use garlic and herbs)
- Do not let pets lick your face or eat off your dishes
- Always wash your hands after using the bathroom
- Wash your hands after working in the garden
- When traveling, don't drink the water

Use anti-parasitic herbs on a regular basis, such as those found in colon cleanse or the anti-parasite formula

Treatment: Anti-Parasite Formula (page 218), Black Walnut hulls, Clove, Wormwood, Quassia, Colon Cleanse, Liver-Gallbladder Formula and Colon Detox. These herbs can be taken in either capsule or tincture form. Six dropperfuls of anti-parasite herbs in tincture (6 to 8 dropperfuls) or 12 to 16 capsules Foods such as pumpkins seeds, garlic, onions and pickles are anti-parasitic. Yogurt is helpful in maintaining and restoring healthy intestinal flora.

PLAGUE - Bacteria (Fleas/Coughing)

Definition/Diagnosis: Plague is a general term for an epidemic of an infectious illness as well as the disease caused by a specific bacteria. It is unfortunate that we have to worry about biological terrorism, but its a reality that could occur. The medical distribution of antibiotics or antidote serums for a massive outbreak is unlikely. I admonish each family group to have an emergency supply of herbal remedies to combat these infectious diseases. Our bodies are capable of fighting infectious illnesses, even the most virulent. The key is to boost the bodies immune system.

"The Plague" is caused by the bacteria Yersinia pestis, that infects wild rodents in many parts of the world. Epidemics occur when domestic rats become infected and spread the disease to man. Bubonic plague is transmitted by infected fleas, while pneumonic plague is spread directly to other people by coughing. Plague is accompanied by fever, enlarged lymph nodes (bubonic plague) and less commonly pneumonia (pneumonic plague). As history attests, the outcome can be fatal.

Treatment: Anti-Plague Formula - 1 Tbs. each hour for the next 3-5 days, until recovered or until instructed by your health care providers. Use the Cold Sheet Treatment as prescribed. Use SuperNutrition 2 to 3 times daily. Use Immune Boost Formula hourly. Avoid exposure and use these same herbs for prevention.

RABIES (Animal Bite)

Definition/Diagnosis: Rabies can be transmitted by many species of mammals namely skunk, bat, fox, coyote, raccoon, bobcat, wolf and to lesser degrees dogs or cats. An attack by a wounded animal is cause for concern. Animals whose bites have never caused rabies in humans in the U.S. are cow, sheep, horse, rabbit, gerbil, chipmunk, squirrel, rat, and mice.

Contaminated saliva or blood of an infected animal if it comes in contact with a break in the skin or mucous membrane can possibly transmit the disease. Incubation period in humans is one to two months. Rabies is a vicious disease that is fatal once it develops clinical symptoms.

Treatment: Medically rabies is treated most effectively with immune globulin protein and a vaccine (human diploid cell vaccine -HDCV) injected into the shoulder on days 0, 3, 7, 14, and 28. If tested positive for rabies (the animal will test positive, not the patient until it's too late), then the medical treatment is advised. If absolutely unavailable, treat aggressively with immune boosting herbs, Cold Sheet Treatment and diet.

RELAPSING FEVER (Body lice/tick)

Definition/Diagnosis: This bacterial infection is spread by body lice in Asia, Africa and Europe, or by ticks in the United States, Asia, Africa and Europe. Symptoms occur 3 to 11 days from contact with the tick or louse (one lice), beginning with an abrupt onset of chills, headache, muscular pains and sometimes vomiting. A rash may appear and small hemorrhages appear under the skins surface. The fever remains high for 3 to 5 days (104° F), then clears up suddenly. After 1 to 2 weeks a somewhat milder relapse begins. Jaundice (yellowed skin and whites of eyes) can occur during the relapse. The illness again clears, but after 2 to 10 days similar episodes reoccur at intervals of 1 to 2 weeks until the body builds an immunity towards the bacteria. Mortality is generally low, occurring in less than 5% of adults.

Treatment: Prevent with good personal hygiene and speedy removal of any ticks (do frequent body checks). Treat with immune boosting herbal remedies (Anti-Plague, Immune Boost), Cold Sheet Treatment and the Incurables Checklist.

ROCKY MOUNTAIN SPOTTED FEVER (Tick)

Definition/Diagnosis: This is an acute and serious infection caused by a microorganism (Rickettsia rickettsii) transmitted by a hard-shelled tick. This infection is not limited to the Rocky Mountain region. Onset of infection is abrupt, after 3 to 12 days after the tick bite. Fever reaches 103° - 104° F within two days. There is considerable headache, chills, and muscle pain at the onset. In four days a rash appears on the wrists, ankles, soles, palms, and then spreads to the trunk. The rash is initially pink but turns to dark blotches and can even ulcerate.

Any suspected case of Rocky Mountain Spotted Fever should be considered a medical emergency. Do not wait for the rash to develop. Death rate is nearly 20% if not treated quickly.

Treatment: Medical antibiotic therapy cuts the death rate to nearly zero. If medical help is not available, treat vigorously with Anti-Plague Syrup (1 Tbs. hourly - 12 to 16 times daily). Perform the Cold Sheet Treatment and Follow the Incurables Checklist.

TAPEWORMS (parasite)

Definition/Diagnosis: There are three species of tapeworm that infect humans. All three infect people as a result of eating undercooked meat of the infected animal (beef, pork, fish). Beef tapeworms can be huge growing up to 30 feet inside the human host. They are common in Mexico, South America, Eastern Europe, the Middle East and Africa. Symptoms can include stomach pain, weight loss, and diarrhea. Often the infected person is unaware of the tapeworms.

Pork tapeworms generally result in vague abdominal complaints and are common in South America, Eastern Europe, Russia and Asia. A complication of this disease is cystocercosis. When a person drinks water infected with the larvae, the tapeworm larvae penetrate the human intestinal wall, which invades the body tissues (frequently the muscles and the brain). As they mature they form cystic masses which after several years degenerate producing local inflammatory reactions that can result in convulsions, visual problems or mental disturbances.

Fish tapeworm occurs worldwide. Usually there are no symptoms. The worm's tendency to absorb Vitamin B-12 may cause pernicious anemia in the person.

Diagnosis is often made by finding a piece of the worm after a bowel movement.

Treatment: It is really unlikely that many of us have escaped parasitic infections. Treat with anti-parasite herbs such as black walnut hulls, wormwood, cloves, and anti-parasite formula, page 218. Foods such as pumpkin seeds, garlic, onions and pickles are also anti-parasitic.

TETANUS - Lockjaw (Bacteria)

Definition/Diagnosis: Tetanus is caused by the bacteria Clostridium tetani. Most cases occur from exposure to tetanus from minor wounds such as blister or paper cuts rather than a rusty nail or barbed wire. Onset is gradual with an incubation period of 2 to 50 days (it's usually 5 to 10 days). The earliest symptoms are stiffness of the jaw which is followed by a sore throat, stiff muscles, headache, low grade fever, and muscle spasms. As the disease progresses, the patient is unable to open the jaw and the facial muscle may be fixed in a smile with elevated eyebrows. Painful muscle spasms of the whole body are set off with minor disturbances such as a cool draft, noises, or someone jarring their bed. Death from loss of respiratory muscle function may result. This disease, if it is allowed to progress, is frequently fatal.

Treatment: Use a plantain poultice over the affected wound (usually a puncture wound). Use lobelia tincture 4-10 drops every hour until jaw relaxes and opens. Boost the immune system with Immune Boost (page 230) and Anti-Plague Formula (page 219). Juicing and the Health Promoting Diet (page 243) should be adhered to. Don't neglect medical care.

THROAT - Infection, Sore (Bacteria/Virus)

Definition/Diagnosis: The most common cause of a sore throat is a viral infection (80%). Antibiotics will not help this. The only type of sore throat to be concerned about is a Strep infection. With a bacterial (Strep) infection there will be a splotchy coating over the red tonsils or back portion of the throat and the throat will be very sore. Lymph node will be swollen in both a bacterial as well as viral infection.

Treatment: Spray or squirt Immune Boost on back of throat. The Echinacea in the Immune Boost will cause a numbness in the throat relieving much of the soreness. Gargle with Herbal Tooth Powder made into a tea. Apply Deep Heat on the outside surface of the neck/throat for relief. Take 1/2 tsp. of hot/garlic honey every 1/2 hour (4 cloves garlic, 1 Tbs. Honey, 1/4 tsp. Cayenne). Do not eat or drink afterward. The garlic is anti-bacterial and will kill the streptococcus bacteria. The cayenne will increase the circulation to the area and the honey will stick everything in place.

Take Immune Boost or Anti-Plague Formula as recommended by your healthcare practitioner.

Make a tea of 1 Tbs. licorice, 1 Tbs. Hyssop, 2 Tbs. Slippery Elm, 1 Tsp. Wild Cherry. Also drink Yarrow tea.

TICK PARALYSIS (Tick)

Definition/Diagnosis: Five species of tick in North America produce a neurotoxin in their saliva that can paralyze its victims. Most cases are from the Pacific Northwest, the Rocky Mountain states and the southern states. Spring and Summer are the high risk seasons.

The toxin is usually carried by an engorged, pregnant tick. Symptoms begin from 2 to 7 days after the tick begins feeding. Throughout the ordeal the patient's mental function is left intact. Symptoms start as weakness in the legs which progressively moves up until the entire body is paralyzed over several hours to days. At times the condition presents as ataxia (loss of coordination) without muscle weakness. The diagnosis is made by finding an embedded tick. After removing the tick, symptoms resolve in hours to days, rarely longer. Untreated tick paralysis can be fatal in 10% to 12%.

Treatment: Find and remove the tick. Tick paralysis only occurs when the tick has gorged itself on you and a regurgitated toxins in to your bloodstream. Follow the Incurables Checklist to ensure a speedy recovery.

TRICHINOSIS (Parasite)

Definition/Diagnosis: Trichinosis is caused by eating improperly cooked meat infected with the cysts of this parasite. It is most common in pigs, bears (especially polar bear), and some marine mammals. Nausea, diarrhea and intestinal cramping may appear in 1 to 7 days after ingestion. Swelling of the eyelids is very characteristic on the 11th day. Afterwards muscle soreness, fever, pain in the eyes and subconjunctival hemorrhage (page 110) develops. If enough contaminated food is eaten, trichinosis can be fatal. Most symptoms disappear in 3 months.

Treatment: Treat for parasites, see page 172. Use herbal pain formula, page 233. Cold Sheet Treatment and Incurables Checklist will speed the recovery.

TONSILLITIS (Virus/Bacteria/Allergy)

Definition/Diagnosis: The tonsils are an important part of our immune system. The tonsils are an aggregation of lymphoid tissue and are the only place where B-cells (a type of white blood cell) can make anti-bodies against Polio. Rarely if ever should they be removed. Most often the tonsils become inflamed due to a virus or allergies.

Treatment: Garlic (fresh - it must be fresh) six cloves daily is effective against both gram positive and gram negative bacteria. Use Garlic/Honey/Cayenne remedy see page 177. Also 1/2 cup of strong tea made from 3 parts Mullein, 1 part Lobelia in a decoction(see instructions page 210). Soak a cloth with this decoction and wrap the throat, then cover with plastic and a hot water bottle. Drink as much red raspberry tea as possible. 1 gallon in 24 hours. Drink 1/2 cup of Mullein/Lobelia tea morning and Evening. Use Immune Boost and Anti-Plague formula. Both Immune Boost and Anti-Plague contain garlic which are very helpful for the tonsils. If the patient experiences other allergy type symptoms and they have a history of allergies, use an allergy syrup. (Astragulus, nettles, marshmallow tinctured then made into a glycerin extract, see page 218).

TUBERCULOSIS - T.B. (Bacteria)

Definition/Diagnosis: Referred to as "consumption" in the old literature (fiction and non). This infection is caused by one of two bacteria, Mycobacterium tuberculosis and M. bovis. It results in a very chronic illness that can lie dormant for many years only to return. This disease is on the rise both in the U.S. and worldwide. It is spread by breathing infected droplets or by consuming infected milk or dairy products such as butter.

The active disease usually develops within a year of contact. The early symptoms are cough, fever, night sweats, fatigue and weight loss (that is gradual). The cough may produce small amounts of green or yellow sputum. As the disease progresses, more sputum is produced until it is streaked with blood. One of the classic symptoms of T.B. is waking up in the night drenched in a cold sweat that is so profuse that sheets or nightclothes need to be changed. This sweat is caused by the subsiding of a low-grade fever that is not readily apparent to the person. Tuberculosis usually infects the lungs, but it can spread throughout the entire body causing neurologic damage (paralysis), bone infections, or infections in the brain, bladder, kidney or heart.

Treatment: This low grade fever, wasting disease can be treated with the Incurables Checklist, cold sheet treatment, immune boosting herbs as well as an herbal tea made of equal parts comfrey root, mullein, chickweed, marshmallow root, and lobelia. Make into a tea and drink 3 to 5 cups daily.

TULAREMIA - Rabbit Fever; Deer Fly Fever (Tick/Fly/Mosquito)

Definition/Diagnosis: This disease can be contracted through exposure to ticks, deer flies, or mosquito's. It is also possible to have cuts infected when working with the pelts, or eating improperly cooked infected rabbits. Similarly, muskrats, foxes, squirrels, mice and rats can spread the disease. Stream water can become contaminated by these animals. When a wound is involved an ulcer appears and the lymph nodes become enlarged(first near the site of infection then spreading throughout the body). Pneumonia normally develops. This disease typically lasts 4 weeks if untreated. If treated mortality is almost zero, untreated from 6% to 30%.

Treatment: Use anti-plague syrup (1 Tbs. 12 to 16 times daily), perform the Cold Sheet Treatment and follow Incurables Checklist. Drink the tea described under tuberculosis.

TYPHUS - Typhoid Fever (Flea)

Definition/Diagnosis: This worldwide disease is spread through infected rat flea feces. After an incubation period of

6 to 18 days (usually around 10 days), shaking chills, fever and headache develop. There is a tendency to diarrhea and nosebleeds. The stools seem to be a pea soup color. At times there could be constipation and a slight congestion of the lungs. A rash (small, slightly elevated, rose-colored spots) forms primarily on the trunk, but fades fairly rapidly. The fever lasts about 12 days. This is a mild disease and fatalities are rare.

Treatment: Prevention is geared toward rat and flea control. Boost immune system with echinacea, garlic, Goldenseal, cat's claw or combination formulae such as Immune Boost and Anti-Plague Syrup. Drink hot yarrow tea and/or red raspberry leaf tea. Do the Cold Sheet Treatment.

VIRAL INFECTIONS (In General)

Immune Boost and/or Anti-Plague Syrup. Cold Sheet Treatment. Drink copious amounts of herbal tea and carrot juice (this means one gallon in 24 hours).

Refer to Boosting the Immune System Naturally on page 246.

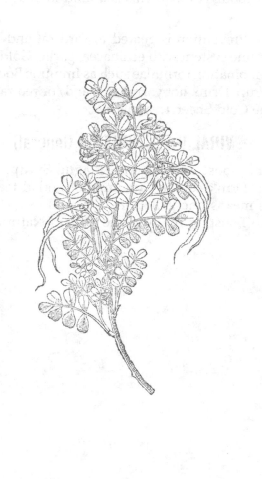

Chapter 12

BITES & STINGS

BITES - Animal

Treatment: Wash the wound immediately with water to flush out the animal's saliva. Then clean the wound for at least five minutes with plenty of soap and water. Rinse thoroughly, gently pat the area dry. Apply Herbal Antiseptic tincture, then a healthy amount of CTR ointment. Cover with a clean dressing. Begin giving the victim Immune Boost - 1 dropperful each hour.

Consult a doctor as soon as possible. He can treat the wound more effectively and decide what measures are necessary to guard against rabies and tetanus.

If the bite is from an unknown dog, cat, or other animal, call the police to try to have the animal caught and observed for rabies. If the animal disappears, or if observation shows that it has rabies, the victim may need anti-rabies injections.

BITES - Human

Definition/Diagnosis: Human bites are usually due to accidents such as falling and puncturing the flesh with teeth. Bites within the persons own mouth seldom become infected. Human bites to any other part of the body have the highest rate of becoming infected as compared to other wounds.

Treatment: Scrub vigorously with soapy water and herbal antiseptic. Pick out any broken teeth or other debris. Use a vacuum extractor (such as the Extractor™ used in snake bites) for 20-30 minutes over the wound. Begin the application of hot, wet compresses as described under puncture wounds (page 198). Herbs to draw out poisons can be made by combining Colon Detox Powder (see page 223) and Immune Boost (page 230) into a paste and applying to the area. Bites to the hand are the most serious and may require attention from a hand surgeon.

BITES- Ant, Chigger, Mosquito

Treatment: Wash the affected parts with soap and water. The object here is to draw the poisons from the bite out of the skin. Apply a paste/poultice of Colon detox mixed with Immune Boost. A poultice made of fresh plantain leaf is very effective. You may also use baking soda and a little water. Leave the poultice on until it dries. You may need to repeat the procedure. Chiggers like to attach themselves to their victim. It takes an hour or more for chiggers to attach themselves firmly. Scrubbing with a brush and soapy water promptly after exposure should remove them. If there is swelling, applying ice or an ice pack will help.

An allergic reaction to ant bites can be serious, occasionally fatal. Begin treating with immune boost and allergy syrup - 1 dropperful of each every ten minutes as you rush them to a hospital emergency room or call 911. Use lobelia tincture to help with breathing. - 5 to 20 drops every 10 minutes or as needed.

1. Apply poultice of Colon Detox and Immune Boost.
2. One tsp. Lavender essential oil with one Tbs. vegetable oil.
3. Plantain poultice
4. Sliced or grated onion used on a bite is also effective.
5. Insect Repellent - 2 oz. Vegetable oil 1/4 tsp. Citronella essential oil, 1/8 tsp. cedar or rose geranium essential oil.
6. Immune boost applied directly to eruptions is known to take the itch away immediately.
7. Other helpful herbs are Aloe vera, Marigold, Comfrey, Elder flower leaves.

POISONOUS SPIDERS and SCORPIONS

Treatment: Treat similarly as for poisonous snake bites.

1. Have person lie down and remain calm; cover them with a blanket, coat, sleeping bag, etc. to maintain normal body temperature.

2. Administer Immune Boost tincture. Dose 1/2 -1 oz. at first; next day 1 dropperful 3 times/day. Plantain tincture 1 dropperful 3x/day; Yarrow tincture 1 dropperful 2x/day; Black Cohosh tincture 10 drops 2x/day.

3. If the bite took place within 30 minutes, tie a piece of cloth 2-5 inches above the bite (not on a joint). Tie snugly, but not too tight. Be able to slip a finger under it. This will reduce the spread of poisons.

4. Wash the bite area with clean water and soap. Apply a cold compress while you make a poultice or fomentation of plantain, then apply over the bite area. CTR ointment can be used. Colon Detox mixed with immune boost tincture (made into a paste) put over the area has powerful drawing abilities. Leave on until redness or swelling is gone.

5 If nervous problems occur (fits, depression, crying, short-tempered) use Nerve Calm tincture. 1 dropperful every hour or as needed. For leg cramps, fevers and chills, use horsetail tincture 1 dropperful 3 times/day.

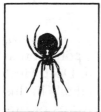 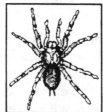 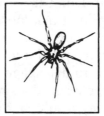 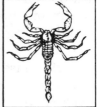

Black Widow Spider, Tarantula, Brown Recluse Spider (fiddler spider) & Scorpion

BITES - Ticks

Definition/Diagnosis: Ticks can cause a potential hazard to anyone in the outdoors because they can transmit many diseases. You should check often for ticks on clothing and exposed areas of your body, and especially your hair on your head and other body parts where they can hide. If you are with someone, have them check your hair on your head about every 2-4 hours. (Run a comb or brush through your hair and then examine your scalp carefully). To help avoid ticks, use Bugs-off oil or Sen-Sei Balm around wrists, ankles, neck and hairline. Tick bites can cause generalized muscular weakness known as "tick paralysis". Any unexplained muscular weakness calls for a body search for ticks or tick bites.

In many locations throughout the U.S. ticks carry the Rocky Mountain Spotted Fever (see page 175). (A sickness with the symptoms of a high fever and red-spotted rash). Lyme disease (see page 170) is another more recent disease carried by ticks. (Symptoms are an expanding, circular, red rash where the tick bite is, flu-like symptoms, a week to a month later, serious heart, joint and nervous system abnormalities occur). The tick that causes Lyme disease is as small as a dot above an "i". It's hard to see, so do a careful search if symptoms appear. Although ticks can transmit dangerous diseases, they usually do not if removed soon after they've become attached.

Treatment/Removal: Try to avoid direct contact with tick on removal. Don't try to tear an embedded tick loose.

First, cover it with a heavy oil (like Deep Heat ointment), petroleum jelly or lip balm to close its breathing pores; often this will cause it to disengage within a half-hour. Deep Heat works well as the insect does not like the essential oils in this product. You may also dislodge it with a few drops of turpentine. If the tick drops off, scrub the area well with soap and water and apply Herbal Anti-Septic tincture. Then apply Colon Detox mixed with Immune boost into a clay poultice to draw out any toxins left in the skin. Internally, take Immune Boost, 1 dropperful 3 times per day.

If the tick doesn't drop off after 30-45 minutes with Vaseline, Chapstick or Deep Heat applied, use clean tweezers to remove.

Tweezers Removal: Turn the tick on its back. Firmly but gently grasp near the head at the point of attachment with tweezers and remove slowly. Work gently so that you don't crush the insect and so that all parts of its head come loose. Make sure to remove entire tick, especially the head and mouth parts.

Apply Colon Detox powder mixed with immune boost tincture. Make into a paste/poultice and apply. Leave on until it dries. A poultice or ointment made of plantain leaves can also be used.

If fever, use yarrow tincture. 1 dropperful 4-6 times per day or until fever breaks.

If the bite become swollen, or if the person has a fever or develops a rash, consult a health care professional.

BITES - Venomous Snake

Definition/Diagnosis: The best treatment for snakebite is prevention. The dangerous venomous snakes in the United States are: the rattlesnake, copperhead, water moccasin and coral snake. More than half of the cases of venomous snakebites occur in Texas, North Carolina, Florida, Georgia, Louisiana, and Arkansas.

If you live or vacation in venomous-snake country, avoid infected areas. If you must enter such areas, wear protective clothing such as mid-calf boots, long pants, and gloves that cover your forearms. Find out in advance of entering snake areas where the nearest medical facility is located. Read up on snakes, their habits and how to avoid their bites.

Treatment: In cases of poisonous snakebite, time is of the essence.

1. Take the person to the nearest hospital at once.
2. Have the person lie down and remain calm and still. Keep the bite below the level of the heart. Remove anything that would constrict (belts, rings, watches, bracelets, etc.).
3. Do not apply ice or any cold therapy. Do not give medication or alcohol other than the small amounts in medicinal tinctures. Skullcap is used to calm the patient and as an antispasmodic.
4. Administer Immune Boost 1 - 2 ounces. Plantain tincture 1 dropperful every 5-10 minutes, Yarrow Tincture 1 dropperful every 10-20 minutes and Black Cohosh Tincture 1-2 dropperfuls 3 times daily. **NOTE: Black Cohosh is a natural antidote for poisons in the system. It has the ability to neutralize the effects of rattlesnake bites,**

scorpion stings, and other poisons in the system.

5. If you have a snakebite kit, apply suction to the bite without making an incision (follow directions in the kit). If you don't have a snakebite kit, use your mouth to suction out the venom. Don't swallow the venom, spit it out, rinsing your mouth out with water often. Continue to mouth suction for at least 15-20 minutes to make sure as much venom is out as possible. (Do not mouth suction if you have open sores in or around the mouth).

6. If you do not have a snakebite kit and the hospital is more than an hour away, apply a constricting band. *Never use the band around a joint (fingers or toes), the head, neck or trunk.* The constricting band should be at least 3/4 to 1 1/2 inches wide. Tie it 2 to 4 inches above the bite, just tight enough to retard the spread of the venom, but not so tight that it shuts off deep-lying circulation of the blood. If the band is properly adjusted, you should be able to slip two fingers under it. With the band in place, proceed with appropriate speed to the medical facility.

7. Wash the bite area with clean water and soap. Apply Herbal Anti-Septic tincture (page 228) over the bite area, then apply a poultice of Colon Detox (page 212) over the bite. If there is swelling, tie a piece of cloth or handkerchief snugly around the bitten limb, 3-5 inches above the bite. If swelling goes beyond this, apply a second band above this one, above the new swelling. Leave the first one on. (Make sure the band doesn't block arterial or venous circulation).

STINGS - BEE, WASP, HORNET

Definition/Diagnosis: Honey bees leave a stinger and venom sack in the victim after a sting. Hornet, yellow jackets, bumble bees and wasps do not leave a stinger and may puncture a person repeatedly. Pain is immediate and is usually accompanied by swelling, redness and inflammation at the site.

Treatment:

1. If anaphylactic shock occurs, it must be treated immediately with epinephrine, such as with an Epi-Pen. Anyone

with a history of anaphylaxis with stings should be prepared with this. If the person is experiencing respiratory distress, lobelia tincture works well to open up the airway. Use 2 to 10 dropperfuls.

2. First remove the stinger and the venom sac as quickly as possible. The venom sac can continue to pump venom into the skin. Just grab the venom sack with your fingers and yank it out.

3. Apply ice or cold water to decrease the pain and inflammation.

4. Colon Detox powder made into a poultice with plantain tincture will quickly draw the venom (toxins) out of the skin. Leave on until the poultice has dried. Bee venom is acidic and can be neutralized by baking soda and water made into a paste.

5. Wasp venom is alkaline and is treated well with apple cider vinegar or lemon juice.

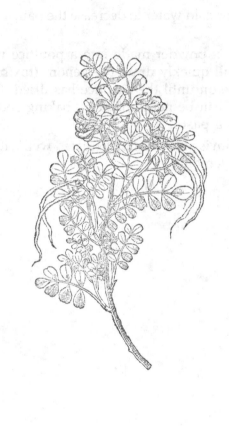

Chapter 13

MOUTH & DENTAL PROBLEMS

DENTAL PAIN - PROBLEMS

Definition/Diagnosis: Cavities may be identified by a visual examination of the mouth in most cases. At times the pain is so severe that the patient cannot tell exactly which tooth is the problem. Tap each tooth until you elicit a strong pain. That's generally the tooth. Dry the tooth and try to clean out any cavity found. Clove oil can be used to deaden the pain. If a filling is lost, again use clove oil as an anesthetic (several drops). Dry the tooth and apply Cavity paste and pack firmly in place. See a dentist as soon as possible. Beeswax can be used in a pinch if you do not have an emergency dental kit. Myrrh gum can also be used.

If a tooth is knocked loose, do not try to push it back into place, you may disrupt the nerve or blood supply. If the tooth is secure at all leave it alone. The musculature of the lips and gums will generally gently push the tooth back into place and keep it there. Use Herbal Mouthwash and Herbal Tooth powder (see page 229) to heal and tighten everything up.

If a tooth is broken with exposed pink substance that is bleeding, showing the nerve, this is a dental emergency. Replace it into the socket immediately. If this cannot be done have the person hold the tooth under their tongue or in their lower lip until you can see a dentist. You must see a dentist immediately. A tooth left out too long will be rejected by the body as a foreign substance.

GUMS (Bleeding, Loose Teeth, Inflammation)

Brush and scrub your teeth and gums with Herbal Tooth Powder and/or gargle with the tea made from this powder. This herbal combination will disinfect, reduce inflammation and tighten up the teeth and gums. Use also Herbal Mouth Wash two to three times daily. Immune Boost or Anti-Plague should be used to prevent or treat any infection.

HERPES (Cold Sores, Fever Blisters)

Immune Boost Tincture 1-2 dropperfuls 3 times daily internally as well as applying directly on fluid-filled blisters. Then apply CTR Ointment (page 224) until the scabbing stage is over. For severe cases you can apply Colon Detox powder over the area before the CTR Ointment. An ointment of lemon balm (Melissa officinalis) is very effective especially if used with the first sign of an outbreak.

MOUTH LACERATIONS

Definition/Diagnosis: Any significant trauma to the mouth can really bleed. The bleeding initially seems to be worse than it is.

Treatment: Rinse the mouth with warm water with herbal antiseptic. This will clear the blood away so you can see where the bleeding is coming from. Bleeding from the lips, gums or tongue usually do not require stitches and generally heal very quickly. Make sure that the area is free from any foreign bodies or debris.

Brush teeth with Herbal Tooth Powder and use Herbal Mouthwash 3-4 times daily (see page 229).

MOUTH SORES (Canker Sores, Aphthous Ulcers)

Definition/Diagnosis: A common cause for mouth sores is rubbing against a sharp tooth or having some dental work. Also eating a lot of sweets can trigger canker sores (aphthous ulcers). These sores can look serious but they are not. These sores can be raised and a kind of orange or whitish in color.

Treatment: Brush your teeth 2 to 3 times daily with herbal tooth powder (page 229). Use herbal mouthwash, myrrh gum, clove oil is a great analgesic (pain reliever). Take immune boost as a mouth rinse. Drink red raspberry tea.

If there is generalized tissue swelling, possible drainage or a whitish cover on the gums, the breath is foul smelling and the gums and tissue of the mouth bleed easily when scraped, it is possible that the victim has trench mouth or Vincent's infection. This is generally caused by poor hygiene. If there is a white exudate over the tonsils, you need to be concerned about Strep throat, mononucleosis, and diptheria. Treat trench mouth by brushing the teeth 3-4 times daily with herbal tooth powder and using herbal mouth wash several times throughout the day.

Fever blisters or cold sores are effectively treated with an oil or ointment made from lemon balm (Melissa officinalis).

TMJ SYNDROME

Definition/Diagnosis: This condition (jaw pain) is spreading in epidemic proportions. Often the pain will radiate into the ear. Often there will be popping or crepitus upon opening and closing the mouth.

Treatment: Taking lobelia tincture 1 dropperful before bed will relax the muscles and often reduce the amount of bruxism (teeth grinding) at night. Warm compresses over the jaw is helpful. For chronic problems CranioSacral Therapy is very effective. Chiropractic adjustments when gently administered and internal massage of the masseter and pterygoid muscles can be helpful. Remember, muscles move bones. Correct the imbalance of the muscles and the bones (temporal mandibular joint) will take care of itself. Do not jump into surgical correction or dental filing of teeth until you've seen a natural health practitioner who specializes in TMJ syndrome. See someone who deals with conservative treatment of the TMJ. It is said that TMJ pain results when the person is supressing fealings that should be expressed. Holding and burying feelings always reemerge in uglier ways. Develop a strategy to properly deal with your stress. Try yoga or meditation practice (see pages 269 and 266).

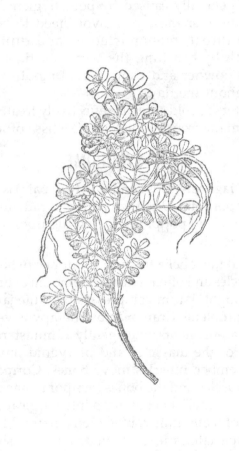

Chapter 14

WOUND & TRAUMA MANAGEMENT

ABRASIONS (Road Rash)

Definition/Diagnosis: An abrasion is the loss of surface skin due to a scraping injury. Often referred to as "road rash". Being a bicycle commuter, recently I have become reacquainted with this affliction, as my left arm and leg can attest. It is not necessary to vigorously scrub these wounds, as the scab will lift out the gravel and debris with it. Be sure and examine the body for possible fractures, dislocations, contusions (bruises), sprains or strains.

Treatment: Clean with soap and water and remove deeply embedded gravel with tweezers. Apply a thick coating of Complete Tissue Repair Ointment to the afflicted area. The CTR will soothe and speed the healing, as well as keep the area from drying out and scabbing over. As life must go on, simply apply a layer of clear plastic wrap to hold the CTR ointment to the wound and prevent the ointment from being rubbed away or absorbed by the bandage. Over the plastic covered wound, wrap gauze or an ace bandage to hold everything in place. Underclothing is often enough to hold everything in place. A couple of times each day add more CTR to the wound. Do not try to remove the old CTR, just keep adding to it. The body will absorb most of the ointment. Allowing the wounds to breath and scab over is fine, although the healing will take a little longer than if you keep it moist with the CTR. Within 6-7 days my recent wounds were completely healed. Very quick healing, I attribute to the CTR ointment. Take Pain Formula for pain, hourly if necessary.

CUTS, SCRATCHES, ABRASIONS

Definition/Diagnosis: Typically if an injury falls into this category, it should be considered "no big deal", however loudly a child may be howling. A little humor mixed with sympathy can go a long way. If this is more than just a minor wound please refer to the sections on wound cleansing, etc. on page 199.

Treatment:

1. To minimize the risk of an infection, wash your hands thoroughly before treating any wound. Clean the skin around the wound with soap and water. Wash the skin away from the wound, not toward it, to avoid contamination.

2. Then, wash the wound itself with soap, flush it thoroughly with water and gently pat it dry. Next you should apply Herbal Anti-Septic Wash to the wound, followed by CTR ointment.

3. Cover the wound with sterile gauze, or the cleanest cloth available, held in place by adhesive tape.

4. Remember that with any wound there is always danger of tetanus (lockjaw); in deep, extensive or dirty wounds, the threat can be serious.

5. Watch carefully for these signs of infection (which may not appear for several days): (1) a reddened, hot painful area surrounding the wound; (1) red streaks radiating from the wound up the arm or leg: (3) swelling around the wound, accompanied by chills or fever.

6. At the first sign of a secondary infection as described above: (1) begin administering immune boost and/or anti-plague formulae; 1 dropperful 4-5 times per day, or 4-5 Tbs./day . (2) Apply a plantain poultice, or Colon Detox-Immune Boost poultice over the site of the wound or infection.

7. Monitor the patients signs and symptoms: pain level, tem-

perature, whether or not the area of infection is close to any vital areas of the body (face, groin, internal organs, etc.). Use your good sense and judgment as to when you should seek professional help.

GANGRENE

Definition/Diagnosis: Burns from fire or acid, frostbite that is not properly cared for, and any wound that becomes stagnant with waste matter in the system can turn into gangrene. Mortification or death to the soft tissues sets in with the failure of the local blood supply. The inflamed or drying tissues are bluish or black in color, and yellow or black spotting with dry gangrene, when the circulation is very poor. People with poor circulation or who have blood that is not clean, run a greater risk of getting gangrene.

Treatment: Colon Cleanse to cleanse toxins from bowel and blood. Take cayenne internally 3-4 times daily. Soak the affected area with Marshmallow root tea, as hot as the person can tolerate it. Apply Deep Heat oil and CTR Ointment.

The renowned herbalist, Dr. Christopher, recommended to make marshmallow root tea (gallons). Soak the affected area for 30 minutes in this tea with 1 tablespoon of cayenne pepper added. Then for 5 minutes put the affected area in ice cold water, then back to the marshmallow tea for 30 minutes. Continue to alternate in this fashion. When the pain has stopped, use a marshmallow tea fomentation (without the cayenne in it).

Use SuperNutrition 2-3 times daily or other comparable green drink.

PAIN

Adequate pain management can be a mixture of proper herbs and attitude. The attitude of both the victim and the person treating is important. A calm professional approach is very important. Pain is a very important symptom that tells you something is wrong. It generally "localizes" or points to the exact cause of the trouble.

An application of cold water or ice can frequently relieve pain. This is important in burns, orthopedic injuries, and skin irritations. Cold can sometimes relieve muscle spasm. Gentle massage and local hot compresses are also effective treatments for muscle spasm. Massaging lobelia tincture or ointment can often relax and break a muscle spasm.

The most powerful pain reliever is opium. When used medicinally it is safe and very effective. Most medical pain relieving drugs are opium derived or based. Natural forms of opium are illegal for general use because of the addictive nature of this herb. Other herbs which can be effective in pain reduction are California poppy, Jamaican Dogwood, Kava kava root, Valerian root, Lobelia herb/seed and Chamomile flower.

PUNCTURE WOUNDS

Treatment: Allow a puncture wound to bleed, thus hoping to let the body clean any bacteria from the wound. A snake bite kit suction device (the Extractor™ can be put immediately over the wound allowing the vacuum to pull for 20 to 30 minutes. Pseudomonis is the predominant germ that infects a puncture wound. Pseudomonis can be killed with acetic acid (Apple Cider Vinegar). Cleanse the wound area with soapy water and apply Herbal antiseptic. Do not tape the puncture wound shut, but rather use a warm compress of plantain, yarrow or catnip tea for 20 minutes every two hours for the next 24 to 48 hours or until it is apparent that no subsurface infection has started. Make these compresses as warm as the person can tolerate without danger of burning the skin. Larger thicker pieces of cloth like a T-shirt work best as they hold the heat longer. Begin using Immune supporting herbs such as Immune Boost.

SPLINTERS (Pieces of Metal, Glass or Wood)

Wash your hands and the skin around the splinter with soap and water. Sterilize tweezers or a needle by boiling them in water or by heating them in the flame of a match and wiping off the carbon with sterile gauze. Loosen the skin around the splinter with the needle, and remove the splinter with tweezers. Apply Herbal Anti-Septic tincture over the wound, cover with CTR ointment and bandage appropriately. Colon Detox/Immune Boost Formula Poultice over the wound can draw out infection or even an imbedded splinter.

WOUNDS - Minor

Definition/Diagnosis: A minor wound is one that is not bleeding excessively or does not require any wound closing procedure such as stitches, staples or taping (butterflies). A wound can be a cut, gash, abrasion, or any other trauma that brakes the skin and causes bleeding.

Treatment: Gently wash out the wound with water that has been boiled or that you know is clean. If slightly bleeding, apply direct pressure for a few minutes. If bleeding does not readily stop, sprinkle with cayenne powder or apply cayenne tincture to stop the bleeding. Cayenne tincture will burn/sting a little more but it will leave the wound cleaner (no excess cayenne powder). Apply Complete Tissue Repair Ointment to the affected area. Apply a sterile dressing if wound is not gaping. If gaping, see wound closure techniques page 201.

Apply Herbal Antiseptic tincture (page 227) to wound to prevent infection.

WOUND CLEANSING

Adequate cleansing is the most important aspect of wound management. Especially when in an isolated or survival situation, the prevention of infection is of critical importance and this can only be assured by aggressive cleansing techniques.

There is an adage in nature: **"The solution to pollution is dilution."** In wound care this means copious irrigation. The whole purpose of scrubbing a wound is to reduce the total number of potentially harmful bacteria. You won't get them all out, but if the total number of germs is small enough, the body's immune system will be able to handle this without an infection setting hold.

Use sterile water for irrigating the wound. This can be done by boiling water for 5 minutes. If this is not possible at least use water that is fit for drinking. Water irrigation is the mainstay of wound cleaning. Use an irrigating syringe or devise something that will allow you to squirt the water with some force. Even a zip lock plastic bag with a hole poked into it can be squeezed so water will come out forcefully. The object here is to allow the velocity of the water to aid in dislodging debris and any germs from the wound site.

You may use a diluted soap solution, but it is not necessary to adequately clean the wound. The best solution to really cleanse and disinfect a wound medically is provodine iodine followed by sterile water. Herbal Anti-Septic formula (page 228) can be used to clean and disinfect a wound. Extended use of alcohol, iodine tincture or mercurochrome are all very harsh and should be avoided except for a short washing. Hydrogen peroxide destroys good tissue as well as germs - do not use this to irrigate a fresh wound. Hydrogen peroxide can be used in cleaning an infected wound.

Besides irrigation, a technique that is used by physicians in the operating room is called "debridement". This literally means the removal of foreign material and contaminated or devitalized tissue from the traumatic or infected lesion. By cleaning the debris or damaged tissue away, healthy tissue is exposed which can heal more easily. Without proper lighting, equipment and training, you will not be able to do a surgical quality job, but you CAN safely come close by rubbing the area vigorously with a piece of sterile gauze or a clean cloth. The rigorous scrubbing action will remove blood clots, torn bits of tissue, pieces of foreign bodies (dirt, rocks, etc.) - all of which have higher bacteria counts. The scrubbing process has to be done very quickly as it is painful and the patient will not be able to tolerate it for very long.

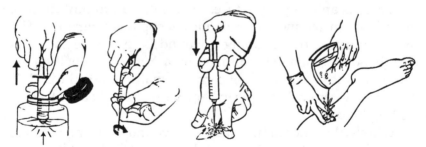

Have everything ready: clean, dry dressing to apply afterward, plenty of sterile water, and an instrument to spread the wound open (a splinter forceps is ideal), and sterile gauze to scrub the wound. If you do not have enough sterile dressings use what you have available. A rough cloth works better at cleaning a wound than a smooth cloth, such as cotton.

Once everything is ready, grab an assistant (someone to

squirt the water into the wound and help comfort the patient), and go for it. If this job is performed well, the final outcome will be great. This part of wound care is far more important than closing the wound. This procedure will be messy and it will hurt but it must be done. Spread the wound apart, blast the water in there and scrub briskly with the gauze pad for 20 to 30 seconds. Be vigorous and thorough. Once completed with this the bleeding will have started again, the blood clots being knocked off during the scrubbing process. Apply a sterile dressing and use direct pressure to stop the bleeding. Usually 5 to 10 minutes will be enough, but apply pressure for an hour or more if necessary. Proceed to wound Closure technique if that is necessary.

Herbal Treatment: Herbal Anti-Septic formula should be used to cleanse and disinfect the wound once it has been scrubbed and washed. Nerve Calm and Pain Formula can be used. 4-8 dropperfuls of each or as necessary. Cayenne can be used internally or externally to stop bleeding. Use Immune Boost prophylactically to prevent infection (2 dropperfuls 3-4 times daily). Apply a heavy amount of Complete Tissue Repair Ointment to the wound to speed the healing. Dress and bandage the wound appropriately.

WOUND CLOSURE TECHNIQUES
(Taping , Stapling, Stitching)

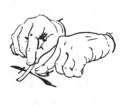

Wounds can be closed using Tape or butterfly bandages. By all means use tape or butterfly bandages if you are able. Taping a wound is very effective for non weight bearing areas (see illustration at right). An improvement to butterfly bandages is the Steri-Strip. Once the wound has been cleaned as indicated above, pinch the wound together and tape shut. You can attach the tape to one edge of the wound and then a different strip to the opposite side and with the two opposing strips pull the wound closed and fasten.

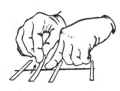

Medically, tincture of benzoin (yes it

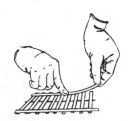

is an herb) is used to enhance the stickiness of tape or wound closure strips. Myrrh or pine resin tincture can act similarly but are not quite as sticky as tincture of benzoin.

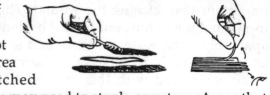

If the tape will not hold (because the area is frequently stretched with movement), you may need to staple or suture. Areas that are highly moving, such as around joints or that are weight bearing like the feet may need stitching or staples. Surgical staples can be very effective and are inexpensive. Staples are not as intimidating as sutures for many. You can make your own butterfly bandages from strips of adhesive tape. Cut the tape into a 3" length (see illustration below). Make four cuts on the sides of either end and fold the sticky sides of the middle together.

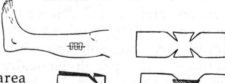

Shaving the wound area has shown to increase the chance of wound infection, even with scalp wounds. If you are going to be closing a wound it must be done within eight hours or not at all. Do not attempt to close any wound after eight hours. Wounds that are torn are said to heal much better than incisions. Remember to use your CTR ointment on the wound, CTR syrup or comfrey tea orally to speed recovery time and insure complete healing.

WOUND INFECTION and INFLAMMATION

Definition/Diagnosis: Lacerations or cuts which have been cleaned and either taped, sutured or stapled together will generally become slightly inflamed. Inflammation is part of the healing process and does not indicate infection, yet the appearance is similar. It is a matter of degree. Inflammation has slight swelling and red color. The hallmarks of infection are: swelling, warmth to the touch, reddish color, and pain. Pus oozing out of a wound is another clue. If the cut has a red swelling that extends beyond 1/4 inch from the wound edge, infection has probably started.

Treatment: The method for treating an infected wound is quite simple. Remove some of the tapes (sutures or staples) and allow the wound to open and drain. **Apply warm, moist compresses of salt water for 15 to 20 minutes every 2 hours.** This will promote drainage of the wound and increase the local circulation, thus bringing large numbers of friendly white blood cells and fibroblasts into the area. The fibroblast (scar tissue cell) tries to wall off the infection and prevent further spread of the germs. If you haven't begun using Immune Boost, begin by using 1-2 dropperfuls every waking hour for the next 3 days. Anti-Plague Formula can always be substituted for Immune Boost or an Echinacea formula. For a wound that is really festering, you may make a poultice of Colon Detox mixed with Immune Boost to assist in drawing out toxins. Plantain in the form of a poultice or as a tincture can be applied to the wound to draw out poisons.

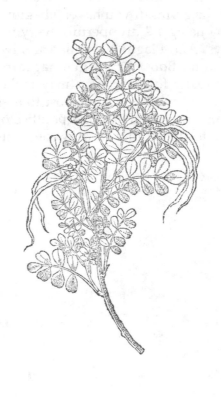

MENTAL WELLNESS

ANXIETY - PANIC ATTACKS

Definition/Diagnosis: Anxiety is more common than usually thought. It can either be acute manifesting as a panic attack when the body's natural "fight or flight" reaction occurs at the wrong time, or chronically manifest as a deep undercurrent of stress and anxiety.

Treatment: Stress can be handled with deep breathing exercises, regular physical exercise, and stress relieving herbs. Herbs such as milk thistle, Bilberry, and ginkgo biloba are useful. Kava kava taken 1-2 dropperfuls 3 times daily for many is just as, or more effective, than anti-anxiety drugs and without the side effects. Nerve Calm Formula 2 dropperfuls 4 times daily. Eliminate caffeine, sugar and alcohol from the diet. Get enough rest. Eat a Health Building Diet (see page 243). Learn to meditate (see "Breath Observation Meditation", page 266). Exercise (non-competitive). Follow the Rules for Getting Well, page 268.

DEPRESSION

Definition/Diagnosis: Clinical depression is more than feeling melancholy or having the blues.

Treatment: Always deal with underlying causes. Exercise can do more for depression than any other form of treatment. Begin a walking or other exercise program no matter how tired or how much you don't feel like it.

· **205**

Nerve Calm Formula - 1-2 dropperfuls 4 times per day to feed & soothe the nerves

Nerve Repair Formula-1-2 dropperfuls 4 times per day to feed & soothe the nerves

Depression Formula - 1-2 dropperfuls 2-3 times per day. Use for 6-8 weeks for best results. St. John's wort is the primary ingredient in this formula.

SuperNutrition - 2-3 times daily

Read inspirational books, meditate daily see page 266.

EXHAUSTION (Fatigue)

Definition/Diagnosis: This is a symptom and not an illness. Always look for the underlying cause. Often it is a matter of re-prioritizing things in our life. The things that matter the most too often are subject to things that matter the least. Most people, with few exceptions, require 7 to 9 hours of sleep per night. Sleep deprivation is not healthy. Look to hormonal imbalances particularly if female or menstrual symptoms are an issue.

Treatment: These are some general recommendations. Double or Triple use of SuperNutrition. Nerve Repair Formula used 2-4 times daily. Build and feed the body with good nutrition rather than stimulating it. Use American Ginseng.

INSOMNIA

Definition/Diagnosis: Habitual sleeplessness or insomnia can be caused by hypoglycemia, muscle aches or injury, indigestion, breathing problems, physical pain, anxiety, stress, grief, depression, jet lag, caffeine consumption, and the use of many drugs including decongestants, anti-depressants, anti-seizure, thyroid and weight loss drugs.

Treatment: Avoid alcohol, tobacco and caffeine. Exercise. Take a hot bath. Nerve Calm Tincture - 1-2 dropperfuls 3 times daily. You may take a large boost of 4-5 dropperfuls before bedtime. Skullcap herb is very effective. A clear conscious does wonders for getting to sleep. Walk barefoot on the grass or bare earth for 5-10 minutes each day.

LETHARGY - Fatigue - Malaise

Definition/Diagnosis: Lethargy, or prolonged tiredness or fatigue, is a non-localizing symptom such as fever or muscle ache (myalgia). Pain, however, is a localizing symptom that points to the organ system which may be the cause of such things as lethargy, fever, or a general ill feeling. Often after a short period of a few days of fatigue - or at times even hours - localizing symptoms develop and the cause of the lethargy can be determined to be an infection of the throat, ear, etc.

Sometimes a chronic condition is the source of the lethargy, such as anemia, leukemia, low thyroid function, depression, low grade infection, or physical exhaustion.

Anemia can be due to a chronic blood loss from ulcers, menstrual problems, lack of adequate formation of red blood cells due to low iron, leukemia and other cancers in the bone marrow, etc. A chronic anemia can be identified by looking at the color of the skin inside the lower eye lids. Pull the lower lid down and look at it. Compare to another person. Normally this thin skin is very orange in color, even if the cheeks are pale, if the color is blanched, white - then anemia is very likely. Another good indication of anemia is an increase in the pulse rate of more than 30 beats per minute in the standing position compared to the lying down position.

Other conditions such as acute mountain sickness can cause lethargy. If nausea is present, think of hepatitis (see page 168). If preceded by a severe sore throat, then infectious mononucleosis (see page 171) may be present. Again, depression can be the cause. In any case proper rest, good nutrition and environment are important.

JET LAG

Siberian Ginseng taken 3 days before and two days after travel will often reduce or alleviate jet lag. With capsules, use 3 per day, tincture 2 dropperfuls per day. Western Botanicals Ginseng Plus will treat jet lag as well as strengthen the adrenal glands.

NERVOUS DISORDERS

Nervous conditions can range from panic/anxiety attacks and nervous ticks/twitches to full blown psychotic episodes. Kava kava is useful for panic attacks and anxiety. St. Johnswort is used for mild to moderate depression. Skullcap for insomnia. Elder Flower tea for twitches and ticks in the eyelid. Nerve Calm Tincture - 1-2 dropperfuls 4 times daily.

Alternating hot and cold hydrotherapy (see Healing Soft Tissue Injuries, page 260). Walk barefoot on the grass at least 10 minutes each day. This will remove the excess static electricity from your body. You are literally grounding yourself. Stop all refined sugar consumption. Sweets leach the calcium from the nerves. Wear only natural fiber clothing. Begin an exercise program such as walking.

WARNING
Discard Old Drugs and Keep Others Locked Up

Unlike herbal tinctures, drugs do not last indefinitely. They may lose their potency or evaporate to harmful concentrations, or their components may recombine harmfully. Discard as unsafe any preparation that has changed color or consistency or become cloudy. Especially avoid the use of oil iodine, eye drops, eye washes, nose drops, cough remedies and medical ointments once past their expiration date.

Keep all medications, including nonprescription drugs such as aspirin, Tylenol and ibuprofen, out of reach from children. When discarding drugs, be sure to dispose of them where they cannot be retrieved by children or pets.

Chapter 16

HERBAL PREPARATIONS

Most herbs dried and stored properly will keep for many years. Although they will lose potency with each passing year. Herbs which are extracted and preserved in an alcohol tincture maintain their potency indefinitely when kept out of direct sunlight and extreme heat.

INSTRUCTIONS for PREPARING HERBAL REMEDIES

When you plan for and prepare a fine meal, you would not want to compromise on ingredients. By using the freshest fruits and vegetables, you are assured of the best finished product. You would not consider using old, diseased, infested or moldy ingredients in your cooking. And so it is with herbs. Use only the very best herbs. Herbs should be grown organically, harvested at the peak of their vitality, used fresh or dried properly. Grow your own in your garden or purchase from reputable growers or dealers. Know what you are getting and settle only for the best. Herbal medicine works only as well as the herbs you use. If you settle for poor quality herbs (because you got a great deal on them), then you must be prepared to have poor results. The highest quality herbs need not be expensive, it is really a matter of finding where to buy your herbs. You will pay more for organic, but it is well worth it. Many growers sell top quality herbs that are not "certified organic" even though they are grown organically. The "certified organic" blessing comes at a high cost ($$) and the process is becoming increasingly political. Again know who you buy from.

Teas (Infusions)

An infusion is made from the flowers and/or leaves of fresh or dried herbs. (herbs may be whole, cut or powdered).

Directions: Bring to a boil one or more cups of water and add 1 Tbs. fresh or 1 tsp. dried herb to each cup of water. Remove from heat and let steep 10-20 minutes. Steeping is letting the herbs sit in the pot with the lid on. For extra strength let it steep longer. Strain and add honey, pure maple syrup or stevia for sweetener if desired. Remember: Never boil an infusion.

Teas (Decoction)

A decoction is made from the bark, inner bark or roots of trees and herbs.

Directions: Bring to a boil 1 or more cups of water. Add 2 Tbs. cut-up root or bark to each cup of water. Gently boil for 5-10 minutes, then remove from heat and let steep for 25-35 minutes. Strain and repeat the process with the same herbs. Add both liquids together and sweeten if desired.

A strong decoction is made by gently simmering the tea/decoction until you have reduced the volume to 1/4 of your starting volume. This process is done in making the anti-plague formula.

Capsules

Powdered herbs can be put into gelatin capsules. Vegetarian capsules are also available. While taking capsules for many is easy and convenient, often you miss much of the benefit that herbs have to offer. By actually tasting the herb, a message is sent to the brain which can begin the physiologic response immediately. Digestion begins with the first taste or smell (digestive juices begin secretion). By bypassing the taste buds, you omit this important part of physiology. One exception would be the colon cleansing herbs, because the chemical (active agent) emodin causes the muscular wall of the intestine to contract regardless of taste or neurologic response. Unfortunately, many have developed very limited and picky tastes (if its not sweet, salty or fatty, many don't want anything to do with it). Swallow capsules as you would a pill. Since capsules float on liquid, try tilting your head forward just before you swallow. This allows the capsules to float to the back of your throat making them easier to swallow.

Powders

Some herbs are taken as powders simply mixed into a liquid such as juice or water. This method is good in that you get the whole herb and it is easily digested. SuperNutrition (see page 217) is a powdered nutritional supplement that is best taken as a powder rather than in capsular form. Stirring into the juice is the easiest and most common way to take SuperNutrition. Favorite juices to take SuperNutrition with are cranberry, orange juice, grape juice and lemonade. For some it is an acquired taste, others prefer taking SuperNutrition capsules.

Herbal Enemas

An enema bag should always be included in any survival kit. Always keep one on hand in the home or when traveling.

Directions: Pour 1-2 quarts of luke warm herbal tea (Catnip, Yarrow, Horsetail, etc.) into a clean enema bag. Retain the liquid as long as possible while massaging the bowel area through the abdomen. (lying on a slant board is ideal). Evacuate the liquid when pressure or discomfort occurs.

Fomentation (Herbal Compress)

Directions: Take a piece of natural cloth (cotton, wool, etc.) and dip it into a warm infusion or decoction(tea). Wring it out just enough so it isn't dripping. Place over desired area and secure it with a piece of plastic and tape.

A good example of a fomentation is:

Castor Oil Fomentation

This is used to get rid of hardened mucus in the body, which may appear as cysts, tumors, polyps or to rid the body of inflammation.

Instructions: Soak a piece of wool flannel or baby's diaper in castor oil, squeeze it slightly so that it doesn't drip much, then place the flannel over the part of the body to be treated. Place a piece of clear plastic wrap over the flannel then place a hot water bottle on top. If you don't have a hot water bottle (get one), then you can use a heating pad over a wet towel (clear wrap between the two). You really need to have moist (wet) heat. A hot water bottle is worth the $5.00 - $8.00. Leave all of this on for 90 minutes (a good time to watch a video or listen to music). You will have to refill the hot water bottle a couple of times because it cools rapidly. You can insulate the hot water bottle with towels so that it will retain its heat longer. After the fomentation comes off, wipe the area down (castor oil is kind of sticky). Then massage the area with olive oil in a circular motion (clockwise is best) for 5 to 10 minutes. Repeat this three times per week or as needed. This castor oil fomentation is excellent for any ailment where the liver is congested - which is often the case in many illnesses. This is also very effective when treating appendicitis. The castor oil soaked flannel can be stored in a zip-lock baggy or plastic and used up to 20 times.

Poultice

Directions: A poultice can be made by heating fresh or dried herbs in some water and straining, placing the herbs in a natural cloth and securing with a piece of plastic and tape over the desired area. Or a poultice can be made by chewing, bruising or chopping fresh herbs and placing them directly on the skin or placing in a wet, natural cloth and securing with a piece of plastic and tape over desired area.

Bolus

A bolus is used internally as a poultice for the vagina or rectal area.

Directions: Mix enough powdered herb with olive or coconut oil until it is the consistency of bread dough. Roll into a long roll the diameter of your smallest finger. Cut into one inch lengths and freeze until ready to use. Insert one or two at night before going to bed. Rinse out with douche or enema in the morning.

Tinctures (Extracts)

Tinctures are much more concentrated than teas and can be easily assimilated. They also have a very long shelf life. One drop of a strong tincture is said to be equivalent to one cup of tea. However, often we recommend one dropperful (about 30 drops) of tincture to be taken as a dose. One dropperful is obtained with one squeeze of the dropper bulb. You do not have to try to fill the whole pipette up. Tinctures or Liquid Extracts are best taken in water or juice. They can also be taken straight into the mouth as well.

Directions: Mix 8 oz. dried/cut herb, or 4 oz. powdered herb to 16 oz. (1 pint) of alcohol. The alcohol must be at least 80 proof. Vodka or Everclear brands are recommended. Age for 14 days, shaking the bottle 2-4 times per day, gently mixing the herbs well. Many believe it is best to go by the phases of the moon, starting on the new moon and ending on the full moon. After 14 days, strain and pour into amber glass bottles and cap tightly. Tinctures will keep this way indefinitely with little loss of potency. It is the ideal way to store herbs if you want them to last. If you don't want to ingest the alcohol, simply add your tincture dose to a cup of boiling hot water. The alcohol will dissipate into the air.

Herbal Oils

Herbal oils are ideal for massaging herbs directly into the skin. An alcohol tincture applied to the skin dries and evaporates too quickly, not allowing for maximum absorption into the body.

Directions: Cover desired amount of dried herbs with extra virgin olive oil. Avoid using fresh herbs, as the moisture in the fresh herbs will cause the oil to go rancid more quickly. Keep in a warm place (in the kitchen is usually fine) for 14 days. To speed up the process you may warm on low heat for 1-2 hours, stirring occasionally. (DO NOT BOIL) Strain and press oil from the herbs. Properly prepared oil, made from very high grade extra virgin olive oil, requires no refrigeration. Store in a cool place away from direct sunlight. An oil will last as long as the oil that you used. If you use a high quality extra virgin olive oil, your herbal oil will last two or more years. If you compromise, it will be much shorter. Most oils and ointments sold in stores already smell rancid. Quality is important.

Glycerites

Classically a glycerite is an herbal tincture which uses glycerin as the menstrum rather than alcohol. Typically this type of formula is very weak. Since alcohol really is the most powerful agent to draw the phytochemicals from the plant, I prefer to begin by making an herbal tincture then heating the tincture to allow the alcohol to evaporate off. Usually reducing the liquid to 50% of its original volume is sufficient. Then add enough glycerin to bring your remedy up to its original volume. 50-60% of your finished product should be glycerin. Always use a pure vegetable glycerin. Glycerites are ideal for children and those who do not want alcohol in their remedies.

Ointments

Directions: Make an herbal oil as directed above. Gently warm the oil and add melted beeswax. Plan on using between 1-3 tsp. beeswax to every 1 ounce of oil. To test the consistency of your ointment, splash a little on a cool counter. Test its consistency, then add more oil or wax as desired.

Herbal Baths

The skin is the largest organ of the body. It eliminates at least 2 pounds of toxins a day. It also brings moisture and air (good and bad) back in to the body through the skin. It is important to keep the skin healthy and open as a channel of elimination and respiration. Herbal baths help to open up skin pores and promote perspiration which assists the body during fevers, eliminating heavy metals and poisons from the body. Open pores also allow the herbs to be absorbed directly into the body without passing through the digestive tract.

Directions: Before bathing, brush your skin with a natural bristle brush or loofa sponge. Drink herbal teas (Catnip, Yarrow, Nettle, Raspberry, Peppermint, etc.)

Ginger Bath: Add 2-4 Tbs. Powdered Ginger to warm bath water. Use for fevers, cold/flu, sore muscles, or whatever ails you.

Herbal Sitz Bath: Soak 4-8 oz. of dried herbs or a gallon size container of fresh herbs in cold water for at least 12 hours. (Use Nettles, Yarrow, Horsetail, etc.) Heat up without boiling. Strain and add to bath water. Soak in it for 20-30 minutes. This is great for pregnancy and to speed recovery of any illness.

Mineral Bath: For radiation or heavy metal poisoning. Add 2 pounds of Epsom Salts to hot bath water. Soak for 30 minutes to 1 hour and then drain. Add 2 pounds of Baking soda to hot bath water and soak for 30 minutes to 1 hour. Drink miso soup and/or yarrow tea while in the bath.

Herbal Footbath: Same as herbal baths but use half as much herbs. Soak feet in a large tub.

Syrups: A syrup is made just as you would make a glycerite. Begin by making an alcohol extract or tincture. After the herbs are strained and pressed off, reduce the tincture over very low heat to 50% of the original volume. Then add pure maple syrup, honey or vegetable glycerine to bring the remedy up to the original volume.

*Use fresh herbs whenever possible as they have more strength than the dried herbs.

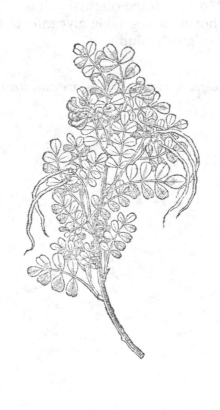

Chapter 17

HERBAL REMEDIES & RECIPES

HERBAL FORMULAE

The formulae contained in this section are here because they work. They have been modified and refined and when made with quality ingredients are very effective. Always use the finest available ingredients. Homegrown and organic are the best. Do not compromise on quality. Pay a little more for quality if you have to. Generally speaking, in preparing these formulae, a part should be a dry or liquid measurement. So when using one cup of a heavy root herb such as wild yam, you will use 1 cup of mullein. If measured by weight, you would need 10 cups of mullein to equal one cup of wild yam.

SuperNutrition™

This naturally balanced blend of organically grown or wildcrafted whole foods is specifically formulated to supply you with Natural Foods Sources of vitamins, minerals, amino acids, enzymes, and essential trace nutrients. All of the ingredients are from the finest organic sources available. Use this product to increase energy, vitality, lose weight or build better health. SuperNutrition will give you the nutritional building blocks to rebuild healthy tissue. This product is recommended to be taken as a powder mixed with juice, however you may also put SuperNutrition in capsules, but you must take 15-20 capsules ("00" size) to equal one dose of powder. Mixing

SuperNutrition with grape juice or lemonade disguise the taste the best. Use with orange juice, cranberry juice, carrot juice or tomato juice. SuperNutrition added to a fruit smoothie is a treat even the kids enjoy. Experiment a little. You will get used to and even enjoy the taste.

Ingredients/Recipe: Spirulina -Blue Green Algae, Chlorella - broken-cell algae, Alfalfa grass, Barley Grass, Wheat Grass, Nettles, Astragalus, Purple Dulse, Beet root, Spinach leaf, Rosehips, Orange Peel, Lemon Peel, Non-Active Nutritional Yeast.

All ingredients are powdered and measured by weight. Equal parts all ingredients except 1/2 part beet. Then 50% of the finished product is Red-Star Nutritional Yeast (we prefer the large flake vegetarian blend).

Allergy Formula

For the temporary relief of allergy symptoms such as runny nose, itching eyes, scratchy throat, sneezing etc. The ephedra in this product can keep some people awake if taken too late in the evening. If anxiety or nervousness results after a few days, discontinue use.

Ingredients/Recipe: Equal parts of the following in powdered form then put into "0" size capsules: Astragalus, Nettles, Marshmallow, Ephedra

A children's syrup can be made using tinctures of Astragalus, nettles and marshmallow, then reduced over low heat and made into a Glycerite. Add a little essential oil such as peppermint, bergamot, or cinnamon for flavor.

Anti-Parasite Formula

This formula is safe and very effective. Parasites are far more common than we would like to think. All of these herbs should be purchased in powdered form and then capsulated in single or double 0 capsules.

6 parts	Black Walnut hull
5 parts	Pumpkin seed
5 parts	Lavendula vera
4 parts	Cramp bark
4 parts	Grapefruit seed and/or peel

4 parts	Wormseed
2.5 parts	Black Current fruit
2.6 parts	Black Current leaf
1 part	Quassia chips
1 part	Olive leaf
1 part	Sweet Annie
1 part	Wormwood leaf

Do not fret if you can't find everything on this list. Do your best with what you can use.

A simpler Anti-parasite formula can be made by combining:

2 parts Black Walnut

2 parts Wormwood

1 part Clove

(Wormwood is very bitter and can be taken in capsule form)

Anti-Plague Syrup

This is our version of the classic immune boosting formula developed by Dr. John Christopher. Use for colds, flu, any infectious illness or "plague". This formula is recommended for any high fever disease that is contagious and can potentially cause death. Not for the timid, only those wanting "Strong Medicine". Take one teaspoon hourly for acute illness or 1/2 to 1 tsp. 3 times per day to boost your immune system.

Ingredients/Recipe:

2 cups Fresh organic garlic

2 cups comfrey root

1 cup each of the following;

wormwood

lobelia

marshmallow root

white oak bark

black walnut hulls

Mullein

Skullcap

Uva ursi
Hydrangea root
Gravel root
64 ounces   *Apple Cider Vinegar*
40 ounces   *Vegetable Glycerin*
40 ounces   *Raw unfiltered honey*

All ingredients are measured by volume, not by weight. Begin by blending the fresh garlic with the apple cider vinegar. Let it tincture for 3 or 4 days before straining. A couple times each day shake this mixture. After the fourth day strain the garlic pulp from the liquid and add it to the glycerin and honey mixture. Please note that this does not require any heat.

Each of the dry ingredients should be soaked and prepared individually. Begin by soaking each ingredient (herb) in 8 ounces of distilled water (32 ounces for the comfrey). After the herbs have soaked for about 4 hours strain off the liquid from the herb. Do not throw away the herb at this point. Add an additional amount of distilled water to the liquid that was strained off to bring your volume up to 8 ounces (16 ounces for the comfrey) Re-combine the herb to the liquid and bring this mixture to a low simmer. Remember each herb is being prepared separately. Simmer for 30 minutes then strain off and discard the herbs. Return the liquid to a stainless steel or glass pan and slowly, over a low heat, simmer the liquid down to 1/4 of its original volume (reduce to 2 oz., 4 oz for the comfrey). With the reduction of each individual herb strain through a fine filter and combine with the glycerin and honey mixture. Once all of your individual strong decoctions have been added to the main mixture (apple cider vinegar, glycerin, honey and garlic), then you are finished. Store in a glass amber bottle in a cool place out of direct sunlight. This syrup can be refrigerated or not. This will make almost 1 1/2 gallons. It seems like a lot (and it is), but for the time and effort, it is worth making it in this volume. It's always good to have plenty of this on hand (just in case or to share with friends).

Be patient, this whole process will take some time but the results will be well worth the effort. This formula will keep for quite a while (2 years - without refrigeration). This formula is labor intensive, but your effort will be well worth it.

Arthritis Tonic

Use for the long term relief of arthritic pain and inflammation. Dietary changes are a must. Eat more fruits and vegetables. Eliminate or greatly reduce consumption of animal products (meat, dairy and eggs). Massage Deep Heat (see page 225) topically for localized joint pain.

Ingredients/Recipe:

2 parts	Cat's Claw
3 parts	Celery seed
1 part	Comfrey leaf
2 parts	Devils' Claw
2 parts	Licorice root
2 parts	Meadowsweet

Make a tincture of the above herbs in 40-50% grain alcohol. Then

2 parts of the above tincture

7 parts of Apple Cider Vinegar (Braggs or Specturm)

7 parts of Raw Honey (local to your area)

Dosage: 1 to 2 Tbs. 2 to 3 times daily.

Brain Circulation - Memory Formula

A great aid for mental fogginess, poor memory, stroke recovery or for an afternoon mental pick-me-up. The herbs in this formula promote more blood and oxygen circulation to the brain. The primary herb in this formula, Ginkgo, is prescribed by more doctors in Germany and France than any pharmaceutical drug. Make into a tincture using 80 proof vodka.

Ingredients/Recipe:

15 parts	Ginkgo leaf
1 part	Rosemary flowers
1 part	Kola nut
1/8 part	Cayenne pepper (the hotter the better)
1 part	Gotu Kola
1 part	Calamus

Calcium Formula

This formula works great for growing pains and muscle cramps. It provides elemental building blocks that are readily absorbable to be utilized by the body.

Ingredients/Recipe:

3 parts	Horsetail
3 parts	Comfrey
3 parts	Oat straw
1 part	Lobelia

Dosage: one to two dropperfuls three times daily, or this tincture can be rubbed directly into cramping muscles.

Colitis Formula

This classic combination is helpful for soothing and healing the bowel or colon afflicted with colitis, Irritable Bowel Syndrome or Crohn's Disease.

Ingredients/Recipe: All ingredients are powdered and the finished product is put in "00" or "0" capsules.

3 parts	Marshmallow root
2 parts	Comfrey root
2 parts	Wild Yam root
2 parts	Ginger root
3 parts	Slippery Elm inner bark
2 parts	Lobelia herb
1/4 part	Cayenne pepper.

Dosage: Take 2 to 5 capsules, 3 times daily or as needed for colitis.

Colon Cleanse™

This formula is used to cleanse, heal and strengthen the entire digestive tract. Colon Cleanse™ stimulates the peristaltic action (the intestinal muscular movement) of the colon and over time strengthens the muscles of the large intestines. Colon Cleanse™ helps to disinfect, soothe and heal the mucous membranes lining the entire digestive system. Colon Cleanse™ aids in digestion, relieves gas, cramps and cleanses the gallbladder and bile ducts, destroying candida albicans overgrowth and parasites, promoting a healthy intestinal flora.

Begin the use of Colon Cleanse™ with 1 capsule during or following the evening meal (some prefer breakfast). This formula works best when taken with food. The following morning you should notice an increase in your bowel action and in the amount of fecal matter that you eliminate. The consistency should also be softer. If there is not a noticeable change in bowel behavior, increase the dosage by one capsule each night until a noticeable change occurs. A bowel movement corresponding with each meal (2 to 3 per day) is considered healthy bowel function.

> **Ingredients/Recipe:** All ingredients are powdered and then capsulated in vegetarian capsules.
>
> | | |
> |---|---|
> | 4 parts | Cape Aloe vera leaf |
> | 2 parts | Senna leaves and/or pods |
> | 2 parts | Cascara sagrada aged bark |
> | 2 parts | Barberry root bark |
> | 1 part | Ginger root |
> | 1 part | Fennel seed |
> | 2 parts | Garlic bulb |
> | 1 part | Cayenne pepper |
> | 1 part | Black Walnut |
> | 1 part | Clove buds |
> | 1 part | Wormwood leaf |

Colon Detox™

This formula is used to cleanse, purify and detoxify the colon, bowels and intestines. Colon Detox™ soothes and strengthens the entire intestinal tract. Colon Detox™ is a strong purifier and intestinal vacuum, helping to draw out old fecal matter from the walls of the colon and from any bowel pockets. Colon Detox™ is uniquely formulated to soften old fecal matter for easy elimination. It aids in the removal of poisons, toxins, parasites and heavy metals. It is also used as a remedy for intestinal inflammation such as diverticulitis, colitis or irritable bowel syndrome. This product is also used effectively for diarrhea or food poisoning.

Colon Detox™ can be used in powder or capsule form. For an intensive colon cleansing (recommended 2 to 4 times yearly, depending on your diet), take Colon Detox™ as directed - 1 heaping teaspoon or 12 capsules, 5 times daily. It is important to take with plenty of water and increase your Colon Cleanse capsules by one to assure 2 to 3 normal bowel movements per day. Taken without sufficient water it can be constipating. Follow this regiment for five or six days.

Ingredients/Recipe: All ingredients are powdered with the exception of the flax seeds which are whole. This is best used in a powdered form but may be put in capsules.

2 parts	Flax seed
2 parts	Apple fruit pectin
2 parts	Pharmaceutical grade Bentonite clay (Aztec Clay)
7 parts	Psyllium seeds and husks (an equal mix of each)
1 part	Fennel seed
1 part	Activated Willow charcoal

Complete Tissue Repair™ (CTR) Syrup & Ointment

This herbal combination is designed to aid and speed the recovery of the bodies connective tissues (bone, tendon, ligaments, muscle and skin). Apply the ointment to wounds, burns(amazing), injuries, ulcer, sores, rashes, cuts, bruises, etc. Syrup helps to heal the body from the inside - out. We recommend syrup for any injury or degenerative bone, muscle or nerve conditions such as osteoporosis, arthritis, MS, ALS, etc. We have witnessed miracles with this formula from the regrowth of fingers cut off to the knuckle to severe burns healing without scarring. For severe injuries glob on a healthy amount of CTR ointment and twice daily add more. Do not rub away the old CTR, just keep adding more.

Ingredients/Recipe: These herbs are combined and made into an oil. Use only the finest Extra Virgin Olive Oil (spend a little extra and get the very best). A great olive oil will remain fresh for over two years without refrigeration. If water or moisture is introduced, it will become rancid much quicker. Use only dried herbs in making an oil.

6 parts	Comfrey root
1 part	St. John's wort

1 part   *Lobelia*
6 parts   *White Oak bark*
3 parts   *Marshmallow root*
3 parts   *Mullein*
3 parts   *Black Walnut bark*
3 parts   *Gravel root*
2 parts   *Wormwood*
1 part   *Skullcap*
2 parts   *White Willow bark*
1 part   *Horsetail*

Cover all of these herbs with Olive oil. As moisture of the oil is absorbed into the herbs add more oil so that you have 1-2 inches of oil above the herb. Ointment- extra virgin Olive Oil, in a base of pure beeswax (see page 214). Syrup - extracted in USP grade grain alcohol and preserved in Pure vegetable glycerin (see page 213-215).

Deep Heat Formula (oil)

Eases muscle soreness, soothes Sprains and Strains, Reduces inflammation of bursitis and tendonitis and relieves arthritis pain. Massage directly into the body for warming & cooling relief. Used for arthritis, bursitis, tendonitis, any ache or pain of the muscle or joint. Very potent and powerful when used in concert with Hot and Cold Hydrotherapy as described in Healing Soft Tissue Injuries section, page 260.

Ingredients/Recipe:

16 oz.   *Wintergreen essential oil*
6 part   *Menthol Crystals*
3 part   *St. John's wort*
3 part   *Lobelia*
1 part   *Arnica flowers*
1 part   *Ginger root*
3 part   *Cayenne pepper*
8 oz.   *Extra Virgin Olive Oil.*

Combine all ingredients in a glass jar. Shake once or twice daily for 14 days. (In phase with the moon is best. Begin on the new moon and strain on the full moon). On day 14 press your oil. A potato ricer works well, or several layers of cheese cloth. Please wear rubber gloves when pressing anything with cayenne. My first experience left me with hands that felt like fire for 3 days.

Deep Heat Ointment

We are so proud of this one. This is a combination of our Deep Heat Formula and our new CTR formula. Rub directly into the muscle or joints that suffer from pain or injury. The ointments consistency is perfect and no worry about spills or drips. Use for Sprains, Strains, Arthritis, Bursitis, Tendonitis, and general aches.

Ingredients/Recipe: Wintergreen essential oil, Menthol Crystals extracted from cornmint, Comfrey root, St. John's wort, Lobelia, Arnica flowers, White Oak bark, Marshmallow root, Ginger root, Mullein, Black Walnut bark, Gravel root, Wormwood, Skullcap, White Willow bark, Horsetail, Cayenne pepper, extra virgin Olive Oil, in a base of pure beeswax.

Ointment contains 1/3 CTR oil and 2/3 Deep Heat oil, add beeswax to thicken into desired consistency (see page 214).

Digestion Aid Formula

The bitter and carminative herbs will increase the digestive juices and reduce gas, bloating and intestinal cramping. Make a tincture.

Ingredients/Recipe:

2 parts	Dandelion root
2 parts	Fennel seeds
2 parts	Ginger root
1 part	Gentian root
1 part	Peppermint
1 part	Licorice root
1/2 part	Chamomile

Essiac Tea

This popular formula is made to the specification outlined by Rene Caisse (Essiac is Caisse spelled backwards), without the endorsement and exorbitant cost. It is a gentle yet powerful blood cleanser used successfully for everything from acne to the worst health problems. All herbs used are organically grown.

Ingredients/Recipe:

6 part	Burdock root - cut
4 part	Sheep sorrel
4 part	Slippery Elm bark
1 part	Turkey Rhubarb root

Female Balancing Formula

This hormone balancing in women relieves PMS and menopausal symptoms such as hot flashes, bloating, anxiety, depression, vaginal dryness, fibroids, abnormal pap smears, abnormal or painful menstrual periods.

Ingredients:

2 parts	Wild Yam root
2 parts	Angelica root (Dong Quai)
2 parts	Chaste tree berries (vitex)
2 parts	Black Cohosh root
1 part	Damiana leaf
1 part	Hops flowers
1 part	Licorice root
1 part	Horsetail herb
1 part	Motherwort herb

Make a tincture preserved in 65% Grain Alcohol. If this is not available use 40-50%.

Headache Formula

Relief for migraine headache pain. Also helpful for many other headaches, increasing circulation to the brain.

Ingredients:

8 parts	Feverfew
8 parts	Lobelia
8 parts	Ginkgo leaf
1 part	Rosemary flowers

1 part	Kola nut
1 part	Cayenne peppers
1 part	Gotu kola herb
1 part	Calamus herb

Herbal Anti-Septic Wash

This can be used diluted as a wash (mix 4 dropperfuls in 4 ounces (1/2 cup) of distilled water). Can be used straight in cleaning wounds or the skin. See Wound Cleaning page 199.

Ingredients:

1 part	Garlic (fresh)
1 part	Goldenseal
1 part	Olive leaf
1 part	Oak bark
1 part	Comfrey
4 parts	Myrrh gum
1/4 part	Tea Tree oil
1/8 part	Cayenne

Tincture in grain alcohol.

Herbal Eyewash

Used for conjunctivitis, cataracts, glaucoma or eye trauma or injury and to clear and build stronger, healthier tissue.

Ingredients:

3 parts	Eyebright herb
3 parts	Bayberry bark
3 parts	Goldenseal root
3 parts	Red raspberry leaf
1/8 part	Cayenne (optional)

Tincture in Grain Alcohol. The cayenne really does improve the effectiveness of this formula. However, I have found that if someone will not use this in the eye because of the heat, then it is better to omit the cayenne.

Dosage: 2 to 8 drops in an eyecup of distilled water. Rinse each eye thoroughly.

Herbal Mouthwash

Used for canker sores, bad breath, cuts in the mouth, bleeding gums, gingivitis, pyorrhea or a gargle for a sore throat. Mix 2 to 4 dropperfuls in a eyecups worth of water (1-2 oz.) Use as a mouthwash. Tincture the herbs before adding the essential oils.

Ingredients/Recipe:

6 parts	Comfrey leaf
3 parts	Horsetail
3 parts	White Oak bark
1 part	Echinacea root
1 part	Lobelia
1 part	Myrrh gum (extracted in 90% alcohol separately then added to the other tinctures)
1/50th part	Clove essential oil
1/10 part	Peppermint essential oil
1/75 part	Tea Tree oil

Do the math and figure it out or go by taste adding a few drops at a time.

Herbal Snuff

For sinus congestion, sinusitis or any chronic sinus problem. Saved many from sinus surgery. Yes, you snuff it up. One pinch per nostril is usually enough. Hold in your nose as long as you can (5 - 10 minutes) before you blow your nose.

Ingredients/Recipe: All herbs are finely powdered

10 parts	Goldenseal root
10 parts	Bayberry bark
4 parts	Horseradish
1/2 part	Cayenne pepper
1/2 part	Garlic

Dosage: use a pinch and snuff up each nostril while holding shut the other. This experience is intense, please do not do this while driving.

Herbal Tooth Powder

Use for gingivitis, pyorrhea, or any other tooth or gum problem or simply for normal tooth brushing. Wet toothbrush, dip into powder and scrub away. You may apply a little toothpaste, wet, then dip in powder. This method is not quite as gritty.

Ingredients/Recipe:

6 parts	Comfrey root
3 parts	Oak bark
1 part	Lobelia
3 parts	Horsetail
1 part	Clove
3 parts	Peppermint

Immune Boost™

This formula works by boosting the number of immune cells and natural chemicals to help fight illness. A very powerful and potent herbal combination to be used at the first sign of any illness. Also available in a non alcohol children's formula. Use in conjunction with the Cold Sheet Treatment and/or Anti-Plague formula.

Ingredients/Recipe:

9 parts	Echinacea angustifolia root
4.5 parts	Echinacea purpurea root
1 part	Siberian Ginseng root
1 part	Pau d'Arco inner bark
1 part	Usnea lichen
1 part	Cat's Claw bark
1 part	Fresh Garlic

Tincture and preserve in 40-50% Grain Alcohol.

Dosage: Acute Illness 1- 2 dropperfuls every waking hour. General use - 1 to 2 dropperfuls 2 to 3 times daily.

A children's version of this formula can be made by substituting the garlic with cinnamon, then making into a glycerite or using pure maple syrup. Reduce as instructed with glycerite preparation.

Kidney/Bladder Formula & Tea

Disinfects the urinary tract, reduces edema(swelling). Use for urinary tract infections, or other kidney/urinary disorders.

Ingredients KB Formula:

2 parts	*Juniper berries*
1 part	*Uva ursi leaves*
1 part	*Horsetail herb*
1 part	*Pipsissewa leaf*
1 part	*Burdock root*
1 part	*Goldenrod flower*

Tincture and preserve in 40-50% Grain Alcohol.

Dosage: 1 to 2 dropperfuls 3 times daily or one dropperful into each cup of KB tea.

Ingredients KB Tea: All ingredients are dried and cut.

2 parts	*Juniper berries*
1 part	*Corn silk*
1 part	*Uva ursi leaf*
1 part	*Horsetail herb*
1 part	*Parsley root*
1 part	*Goldenrod flowers*
1 part	*Dandelion leaf*
1 part	*Orange peel*
1 part	*Peppermint leaf*
1 part	*Hydrangea root*
1 part	*Gravel root*
1 part	*Marshmallow root*

1 teaspoon of dried herb for each cup of boiling water.

Liver Detox Tea

Acts to detoxify the liver, stimulate the digestive system and cleanse the blood, skin, liver and gallbladder. As liver function improves energy will increase. An excellent replacement for coffee.

Ingredients/Recipe:

2 parts	*Dandelion root*
1 part	*All other herbs: Burdock root, Pau d'Arco, Fennel seed, Horsetail herb, Orange peel, Cardamom*

> seed, Cinnamon bark, licorice root, juniper berries,
> Ginger root, Black peppercorns, Uva ursi leaves,
> Clove buds, Dandelion leaf, Sassafras root, Parsley
> leaf or root.

Mix all ingredients together. Use to make infusions and decoctions.

Dosage: 1 tsp. dried herb to each cup of boiling water.

Liver/Gallbladder Formula

These herbs are best known for their ability to stimulate, cleanse and protect the liver and gallbladder as well as rid the body of parasites. Use for any liver concern. Also boost energy.

Ingredients/Recipe:

4 parts   Milk Thistle seed

1 part   each of all other herbs: Dandelion root, Oregon Grape root, Gentian root, Wormwood leaf, Black Walnut hull, Ginger root, Garlic bulb, Fennel seed, Fringetree root. Tincture and preserve in 40-50% Grain Alcohol.

Dosage: 1 to 2 dropperfuls 3 times daily.

Lung Formula

Relieves lung congestion, soothes coughs and eases breathing. This formula has been shown to dilate the bronchial passages and loosen mucus and phlegm so it can be expelled from the lungs.

Ingredients/Recipe:

4 parts   Lobelia herb

1 part   Peppermint essential oil

2 parts   Ephedra herb

1 part   Coffee bean

Tincture the herbs in 1/3 organic raw apple cider vinegar and 2/3 grain alcohol. Add the peppermint essential oil to the finished tincture.

Dosage: 2 drops to 2 dropperfuls in water or juice. This formula is powerful, work into it slowly.

Nerve Calm Formula

This formula is both a sedative and anti-spasmodic designed to relax, sedate and relieve tension and muscle spasm. For insomnia and anxiety. Can be used with children.

Ingredients/Recipe:

2 parts	*Valerian root*
2 parts	*Lobelia herb*
1 part	*each of all other herbs: Passionflower herb, Hops flowers, Black Cohosh root, Blue Cohosh root, Skullcap herb,Wild Yam rhizome*

Tincture and preserve in 65% Grain Alcohol.

Additional **Herbal Muscle Relaxants:** Black Cohosh, Blue Cohosh, Boneset, Brigham tea, Chamomile, Catnip, Cramp bark, Cayenne, Chaparral, Cinnamon, Cloves, Cumin, Elder bark, Elecampane, Eucalyptus, Fennel, Garlic, Gentian, Lobelia, Marigold, Mistletoe, Motherwort, Mullein, Oats, Parsley, Passion flower, Pennyroyal, Peppermint, Pleurisy root, Red clover, Rosemary, Skullcap, Skunk cabbage, Spearmint, Tansy, Thyme and oil, Valerian, Vervain, White poplar, Wild yam.

Nerve Repair Formula

This formula helps to wake up the nervous system. It stimulates the nerves to work better and also stimulates the healing and repair of damaged nerve tissues. Recommended for anxiety, panic attacks, nervous tension and degenerative nervous system conditions. Also excellent for nerve pain such as sciatica or a "pinched nerve".

Ingredients/Recipe:

4 parts	*Skullcap herb*
4 parts	*Oat seed*
1 part	*Celery seed*
2 parts	*St. John's wort flower*
1 part	*Lavender flower*
1 part	*Coffee bean*

Dosage: 1 to 2 dropperful 3 or 4 times daily, or as needed.

Pain Relief Formula

Non-narcotic pain relief, particularly suited for chronic pain.

Relaxes and calms nervous irritation associated with pain.

Ingredients/Recipe:

2 parts	Kava kava
2 parts	Jamaican Dogwood
2 parts	California poppy
1 part	Chamomile flower
2 parts	Valerian root
1/2 part	Comfrey leaf
2 parts	Lobelia herb
1 part	Wild Yam root
2 parts	White Willow Bark

Tincture and preserve in 40-50% Grain Alcohol.

Dosage: 1 to 2 dropperful 3 or 4 times daily, or as needed.

Single herbs used to relieve pain when administered orally. Kava kava, Papavera somniferi, Jamaican dogwood, Chamomile, Valerian root, Lobelia, California poppy, Wild yam root, Catnip, Dill, Flaxseed, Mullein, Skullcap, Skunk Cabbage, Stinging nettle, Wood Betony, poplar buds.

Make a tincture of what you have available to keep on hand.

Potassium Broth - Potato Peeling Broth

This broth is excellent at restoring and balancing electrolyte imbalances in the body. Because of diet and stress our bodies can become overly acidic. Potassium is the great "alkalizer". This broth can neutralize acids in the body associated with muscle cramps and arthritis. Because of potassium's effect on the muscle, imbalance and a lack of coordination are one of the first signs of a potassium deficiency.

Potato Peeling Broth Instructions

In a pot of purified (distilled) water add potato peeling (wash potatoes and skin 1/4 to 1/2 inch deep). Approximately 1/2 of your ingredients should be potato peels. Then add beet tops, celery, onion, garlic and black peppercorns. Simmer on low heat until everything is cooked well. Strain and drink the broth hot or cold. You may lightly salt with Braggs liquid aminos or sea salt. If you don't have everything, use what you've got.

Stone Dissolve Tea

The success of this herbal routine has been documented with pre and post x-rays and has helped many avoid surgery. For kidney stones, gravel, and gallstones.

Ingredients: All herbs are cut and sifted

2 parts	Hydrangea root
2 parts	Gravel root
1 part	Marshmallow root
2 parts	Rose hips

Mix 1/4 cup of dried herb to 1 quart of apple cider, boil for 20 minutes, then strain. You may also use water. Drink at least 2 quarts each day for an active stone, 2 to 3 cups daily for maintenance.

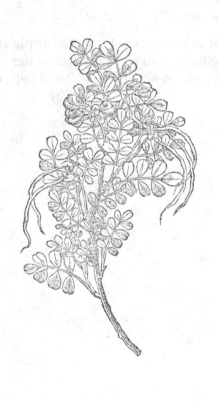

Chapter 18

WHOLE HERB TINCTURES

While many are inclined to use herbal combinations, do not neglect the power and effectiveness of single herb tinctures. As follows are some that you may want to tincture and keep on hand.

Arnica flowers (*Arnica montana*) Use externally for soft tissue injury resultant from dislocations, sprains, cuts, wound healing, bruises, varicose ulcers, and as a throat gargle. Can cause contact dermatitis when used externally, and collapse when taken internally. For external use only. We use this in an oil.

Black Cohosh root (*Cimicifuga racemosa*) Use internally for bronchial infections, menstrual and menopausal problems particularly hot flashes, labor and postpartum pains; arthritic and rheumatic diseases. Excess causes nausea and vomiting. Not given during pregnancy and lactation.

Cayenne pepper fruit (*Capsicum annuum habanero*) Use internally for the cold stage of fevers, debility in convalescence or old age, varicose veins, asthma, and digestive problems. Externally for sprains, unbroken chilblains, neuralgia, lumbago, and pleurisy.

Dandelion root (*Taraxacum officinalis*) Dandelion is a good general tonic. It brings quick relief to chronic inflammation of the liver. Relieves stomach cramps, is a diuretic and helps chronic skin disorders such as rashes, eczema and acne. Use internally for gall bladder, and urinary disorders, gallstones, jaundice, cirrhosis, dyspepsia with constipation, edema associated with high blood pressure and heart weakness, chronic joint and skin complaints, gout, eczema, and acne.

Ginger rhizome *(Zingiber officinalis)* Use internally for motion sickness, morning sickness, indigestion, colic, abdominal chills, colds, coughs, influenza, and peripheral circulation problems. Externally for spasmodic pain, rheumatism, lumbago, menstrual cramps, and sprains. Not for patients with inflammatory skin complaints, ulcers of digestive tract, or high fevers.

Goldenseal root *(Hydrastis canadensis)* Use internally for digestive disorders, peptic ulcers, excess mucus, sinusitis, excessive and painful menstruation, postpartum hemorrhage, and pelvic inflammatory disease. Externally for eczema, ear inflammations, conjunctivitis, vaginal infections, and gum disease. Not given to pregnant women or patients with high blood pressure. Destroys beneficial intestinal organisms as well as pathogens, so it is prescribed for limited periods only (maximum three months).

Horsetail herb *(Equisetum arvense)* Horsetail is most helpful when all other diuretics fail. Use internally for prostatitis, incontinence, cystitis and urethitis. Internally and externally for hemorrhage. Also used for pain caused by arthritis, rheumatism and gout. Can be used internally and externally for leg cramps especially during pregnancy and childbirth. Use for ulcerated legs, itching rash, herpes, hemorrhoids, visual defects, nervousness, nose bleeds, bedwetting, depression, bursitis, bleeding gums, tonsillitis, disorders of the lungs, uterus and stomach and chronic bronchitis. An irritant, best combined with demulcent herbs, and restricted to short-term use.

Kava Kava root *(Piper methysticum)* Use internally for anxiety, nervous tension, genitourinary infections, gall bladder complaints, arthritis, and rheumatism; externally for joint pains. Not given to pregnant women. Excess causes stupor.

Licorice root *(Glycyrrhiza glabra)* Use internally for Addison's disease, as a digestive aid, asthma, bronchitis, coughs, peptic ulcer, arthritis, allergic complaints, and following steroid therapy. Externally for eczema, herpes and shingles. Not given to pregnant women or patients with high blood pressure, kidney disease, or taking digoxin-based medications. Excess causes water retention and raised blood pressure.

Lobelia herb *(Lobelia inflata)* Use internally for asthma, bronchitis, whooping cough and pleurisy as a general nerve and muscle relaxant or to induce vomiting. Externally for pleurisy, rheumatism, tennis elbow, whiplash injuries, boils, and ulcers. When making a tincture of lobelia use 1/3 apple cider vinegar and 2/3 40-50% alcohol. Both the apple cider vinegar and the alcohol will extract different properties from the lobelia that the other won't. A good quality lobelia tincture will cause the back of your throat to feel kind of scratchy for a couple of minutes after taking it. If you don't experience this sensation, you do not have a good product.

> **WARNING:** This herb and its alkaloids are subject to legal restrictions in some countries. Excess causes nausea, vomiting, drowsiness. Not given to pregnant women or patients with heart complaints.

Mint *(Mentha species)* - Mint is calming to the nerves as well as spiritually uplifting.

Catnip flower/herb *(Nepeta cataria)* - Use internally for feverish illnesses (colds & flu), insomnia, excitability, palpitations, nervous indigestion, diarrhea, stomach upsets, and colic.

Peppermint *(Mentha piperita)* - Use for toothache, nausea, colic, gas, headache, insomnia, fevers and dysentery

Spearmint *(Mentha spicata)* - Used for the same conditions as peppermint but especially good during pregnancy when peppermint isn't well tolerated.

Horsemint - This "field" mint is easily available and is good for colds, colic, gas, and diarrhea.

Pennyroyal *(Mentha pulegium)* - Used for colds, flu, fever, jaundice, gas and epilepsy. (pregnant women should not drink more than 1-2 cups of tea a day, and never use the oil).

Mullein leaf *(Varbascum thapsus)* - Mullein is soothing and calming. Breaks up mucus congestion. Use internally for coughs, whooping cough, bronchitis, laryngitis, tonsillitis, tracheitis, asthma, influenza, excess respiratory mucus, tuberculosis, urinary tract infections, nervous tension, and insomnia. Externally for earaches (flowers and/or leaf in olive oil), sores, wounds, boils, blisters, rheumatic pain, hemorrhoids, and chilblains. Use as a skin wash for soothing and easing pain.

Myrrh gum *(Commiphora molmol)* Astringent, antiseptic, and antimicrobial. Increases the WBC activity fourfold. Most effective for sore throats, canker sores, gingivitis. For any mouth, gum, throat or digestive problem. Used to cause the skin to be sticky when using a butterfly bandage or steri-strips. Used in a gargle as in Herbal Mouthwash or as an antiseptic in Herbal Antiseptic Wash.

Nettle leaf *(Urtica dioica)* Use internally for allergies, anemia, hemorrhage (especially uterine). It is kind of like a mild cayenne in its stimulating circulation effect. Use for fatigue or exhaustion. Good for liver, gallbladder, and spleen disorders, headaches anemia, blood disorders, colds/flu, allergies, excessive menstruation, hemorrhoids, arthritis, rheumatism, gout, and skin complaints (especially eczema). Externally for arthritic pain, gout, sciatica, neuralgia, hemorrhoids, scalp and hair problems, burns, insect bites, and nosebleed. Combines well with burdock root for eczema.

Oregon Grape root *(Berberis vulgaris)* Works as an antiseptic and antibacterial. It can be used to lower fevers, for swelling and infected conditions, and as a laxative and intestinal strengthener. It is an antibacterial skin wash and a liver stimulant particularly useful for gallbladder complaints. It is one of the best blood purifiers. Use internally for hepatitis, liver tumor, gallstones, hypertension and cancer chemotherapy. Highly regarded as a liver tonic and detoxifier. Not given to pregnant women.

Plantain herb *(Plantago major)* Use internally for constipation and diarrhea. Externally for poisonous bites and stings. It is Nature's remedy for dog bites, cuts, scratches, wounds, blisters, bee and wasp stings, open oozing sores, and all skin maladies. Use for lung, bronchitis, bronchial asthma and phlegm in the lungs. Use for any skin irritation and inflamed eyelids.

Red Clover blossom *(Trifolium pratense)* Use internally for skin complaints (especially eczema and psoriasis), cancers of the breast, ovaries, and lymphatic systems, chronic degenerative diseases, gout, whooping cough, and dry cough. It is high in chromium which is essential in producing Glucose Tolerance Factor which is necessary in the production and utilization of insulin. Red clover has a calming effect on the whole nervous system and is one of the best herbs to assist in chronic illnesses in both adults and children.

Shepherd's Purse herb *(Capsella bursa pastoris)* Use internally and externally to stop bleeding, especially with heavy menstruation or childbirth, blood in urine, hemorrhoids, nosebleed, and wounds. Also internally for cystitis, and externally for varicose veins. Also for hypertension and postpartum bleeding.

Skullcap herb *(Scutellaria lateriflora)* Use internally for nervous and convulsive complaints, insomnia, irritability, delirium tremens, neuralgia, and withdrawal from barbiturates and tranquilizers. Excess causes giddiness, stupor, confusion, and twitching. Not given in pregnancy.

St. John's wort flowers *(Hypericum perforatum)* Use internally for mild to moderate depression, nervous tension, anxiety, menopausal disturbances, premenstrual syndrome, shingles, sciatica, fibrositis, enuresis in children, and is anti-viral. Externally for burns, bruises, injuries (especially deep or painful wounds involving nerve damage), sores, sciatica, neuralgia, cramps, sprains, and tennis elbow. Not recommended for patients with severe depression and psychosis.

Valerian root *(Valeriana officinalis)* Use internally for insomnia, hysteria, anxiety, cramps, migraines, indigestion of nervous origin, hypertension, and painful menstruation. Excess causes headaches, palpitations, and stupor; extended use may lead to addiction. Externally for eczema, ulcers, and minor injuries (especially splinters). Best on people with cold, nervous dispositions. Not given to patients with liver problems.

Wild Yam root *(Dioscorea villosa)* Use internally for arthritis, colitis, irritable bowel syndrome, diverticulitis, gastritis (esp. in alcoholics), gall bladder inflammation or complaints, Crohn's disease, morning sickness, painful menstruation, ovarian and labor pains, bronchitis, excess mucus, asthma, whooping cough, and cramps.

White Oak bark *(Quercus alba)* Use internally to reduce inflammation, control diarrhea, chronic nosebleeds and hemorrhage. Externally for sore throats, topical herpes, hemorrhoids, bleeding gums, minor injuries, dermatitis, weeping eczema, ringworm, ulcers, and varicose veins.

White Willow bark *(Salix alba)* Salicylic acid - the main active ingredient in white willow bark is known in the medical world as aspirin. It is an excellent remedy for arthritis and for pain relief in general. Mixed with vinegar it can be used to remove warts, corns and "superfluous flesh". Unlike aspirin, white willow does not thin the blood or irritate the lining of the stomach. It is both analgesic and anti-inflammatory.

Yarrow flower/herb *(Achillea millefolium)* Yarrow is a powerful healer and purifier. Use internally for feverish illnesses (especially colds, influenza, and measles), mucus, diarrhea, lack of appetite, gas, nose bleeds, general hemorrhage, muscular pain, varicosities with pregnancy, stomach disorders or bleeding, dyspepsia/indigestion, rheumatism, arthritis, menstrual and menopausal complaints, colds/flu, skin infections, boils and pimples, hypertension, and to protect against thrombosis after stroke or heart attack. Externally for wounds, nosebleeds, ulcers, inflamed eyes, and hemorrhoids. Yarrow was considered by the "old herbalist" a cure for all ills. Prolonged use of yarrow may cause allergic rashes and make the skin more sensitive to sunlight.

Yellow dock root *(Rumex crispus)* Use internally for chronic skin diseases, jaundice, constipation (especially associated with skin eruptions/ acne), liver disorders, and anemia. High source of organic iron. Excess may cause nausea and dermatitis.

Use herbs that are available and are indigenous to your ethnicity and region. As follows are alternative herbs for various purposes.

Chapter 19

PROGRAMS & PROTOCOLS

A HEALTH PROMOTING DIET

The foods we eat and our diets are woven so deeply into our emotional make-up that lasting change occurs as a result of strong emotions. Most of us are aware that we don't eat as well as we could. Before you decide to improve your diet, first decide why you are doing it. I caution you that to change for a negative reason ("so I don't die, because I want to get my blood cholesterol down") are poor reasons. Rather look to the positive rewards of adopting a new eating lifestyle ("to enjoy my health and grandchildren for years to come, so I can enjoy physical activity, so I can better fulfill my life mission with more vibrant energy"). The way we look at change really is important.

So What Should I Eat?

When you are very ill, the best thing you can do is to nourish the body without putting any undue stress on the digestive system. When acutely ill or injured a diet consisting of fresh raw juices, such as carrot juice is best. You may drink a gallon per day for several days or weeks.

The next level of diet would be to eat a raw foods diet consisting of raw fruits, vegetables, nuts and seeds. Raw foods are easily digested and assimilated.

Your normal diet and primary staples should consist of predominately whole grains (starches) with the addition of vegetables, fruit, nuts and seeds. Of course, there are other things you will eat, but 90 - 95% should be whole grains, vegetables, fruits, nuts and seeds.

Eat a diet centered around whole grains (rice, wheat, oats, millet, rye, spelt, corn, amaranth, buckwheat, barley, couscous, quinoa, kamut, etc.), potatoes, whole grain pastas, beans, lentils, seeds and nuts. Emphasize a variety of organic whole grains, legumes and vegetables and de-emphasize flour products like breads and muffins. Eat several pieces of fresh fruit each day, especially before noon. Eat fruits and vegetables fresh and in season whenever possible. Of course, organic is best and many local farmers markets carry organic and some organic growers even will deliver weekly.

Chew your food thoroughly (to the consistency of applesauce). Eat slowly (set your fork down between bites). Drink plenty of water (8 oz. 10 minutes before your meal is a good habit). Drink at least 8 glasses of water, fresh juices or herbal teas (64 oz. or 1/2 gallon) each day. Increasing consumption by one glass of water for every 25 pounds you are overweight will help you lose unwanted pounds. Eat high-quality, whole, unprocessed food. Remain open to change, experimentation, growth and new recipes.

If you crave sugar and sweets take bitter herbs daily. Bitter herbs such as dandelion, gentian and oregon grape root stimulate bile production and will decrease the cravings for sugar.

Some Foods to Avoid

Salt: Change from processed table salt to sea salt. We like Celtic Sea Salt. When your body craves salt, it is asking for all of the minerals naturally found in salt from the sea, not just refined sodium chloride with iodine. Sea salt is balanced with essential minerals and trace minerals needed for good health. Using natural sea salt is a healthy choice.

Refined Flours & Sugars: Avoid these as they are constipating, mucus forming and do not have the nutritional value of whole foods. As you adapt your diet to whole food sources these refined products will begin to lose their appeal and strong emotional draw.

Milk, Dairy, Eggs: Use very sparingly if at all. There are so many natural health substitutes that you'll hardly miss them. These foods create a lot of mucus in your digestive tract and are constipating. Stop using milk as a beverage. Substitute fruit juices for your children. Drink more water, juice and herb teas. Try soy, rice or almond milk on cereals and in cooking. One of the main concerns regarding the milk, cheese and eggs we purchase is that they're contaminated with hormones and antibiotics (many scientists suggest that minute trace amounts of antibiotics in our food supplies are responsible for the drug resistant infections that are appearing). If you use cheese, use only as a condiment to garnish foods. Hard cheeses such as parmesan and Romano are healthier choices than soft cheeses (American, Jack or Cheddar). Use eggs from organically fed free-range chickens. Never, never use margarine, it is damaging to your arteries. If at all, use real butter, very sparingly. Try olive oil as a butter substitute. Use olive oil on your next baked potato.

Meat: Our definition: anything that has a face. Use it sparingly if at all. Hormone, pesticides, herbicides, and many drug residues and contaminants are found in our meat supplies. Meat, if used, should be used to garnish and add flavor to your food, not as the main course. If you do eat meat on occasion, cold water fish, like salmon, is best. Many healthfood stores carry meat from organically fed, chemical-free animals.

Obvious Unhealthy Products: Eliminate completely; soda pop, tobacco, coffee, black/green tea (the types with caffeine), alcohol, and foods with artificial preservatives, flavors, colors, etc. Read the labels on the products you buy. If it has a chemically sounding name, then be suspicious of its health value.

Supplements: As a general overall nutritional supplement we recommend one of the many "Green drinks". Whole food supplements are the only types of supplements that should be taken. By isolating and concentrating active ingredients you create a drug, even though it may have started as an herb. Medicinal herbs in general can be considered as concentrated foods. This book offers many herbal remedies designed to assist your bodies natural healing abilities restoring you to your optimal health. The body was designed to utilize nutrients as they are made by nature. Natural wholefood herbal supplements are a better choice than those synthetically made by man in a laboratory.

One of the secrets to a healthy diet and lifestyle is recipes. Some books we use and recommend are: *Vegetarian Cooking for Everyone,* by Deborah Madison, *The McDougall Program,* by John McDougall, M.D., and *Diet for a New America,* by John Robbins. Peter D'Adamo's book on eating according to your blood type will help you identify foods that you may be sensitive or allergic to. *Vegetarian Times* magazine is also a valuable resource for recipes and articles.

Remember, it's not what you eat some of the time, but what you eat most of the time that will ultimately determine your health. Often I find myself caught in a negotiating process with a patient as to what they can and cannot eat. Remember, we are each free to choose our actions, but not the consequences of those actions. Learn to be honest with yourself and your eating habits. And please don't expect to escape the consequences, either good or bad, of your eating choices. If you are unwilling to make healthy changes, then become aware of the health risks involved.

Boosting the Immune system Naturally

The immune system is perhaps one of the most complex and fascinating systems of the body. The immune system's prime function is protecting the body against infection and the development of cancers or abnormal cells. Conditions such as colds, influenza, allergies, asthma, mononucleosis, fibromyalgia, chronic fatigue syndrome, auto-immune disorders such as Multiple Sclerosis (MS) and many cancers are all directly associated with a weakened immune system. A primary key to recovery is Strengthening the Immune System.

Stress causes an increase in the adrenal gland hormones which inhibit the immune system. Prolonged stress can leave a person susceptible to infections, cancer and other illnesses. Inadequate rest can be the greatest strain on the immune system. During sleep and deep relaxation powerful immune enhancing compounds are released and many immune functions are greatly increased. Good quality sleep and relaxation to counteract stress are vital for healing and a healthy immune system.

Eating highly sweet and sugary foods reduce the white blood

cells ability to destroy bacteria. White blood cells are the immune systems fighting soldiers designed to keep foreign invaders (germs, bacteria, virus, etc.) at bay and the local riffraff (abnormal cells) under control. 100 grams of sugar in the form of glucose, fructose, honey and fruit juices (simple sugars or carbohydrates) significantly reduces the immune response. In contrast, eating starches (complex carbohydrates) had no negative effect. The average American consumes 150 grams of refined sugar in their diets each day. The inescapable conclusion is that most Americans have a chronically depressed immune system. Consuming simple sugars (even orange juice) during an infection is detrimental to the immune response.

Obesity, diabetes, high cholesterol and high triglycerides also inhibit various immune functions. Consuming alcohol increases susceptibility to infections.

Several herbs such as Echinacea, Garlic, Goldenseal, Cat's Claw, and Pau d'Arco have shown to enhance the body's inherent immune mechanisms. These herbs are effective against viral as well as bacterial infections. Studies and research have also demonstrated that Vitamins A, beta-carotene, Vitamin C, Zinc, Iron, and pyridoxine (Vitamin B-6) all enhance and boost the body's immune system.

THE COMMON COLD IS THE CURE

For years scientists and researchers have tried to discover "the cure" for the common cold. It has not been found and never will be, for one simple reason: The Common Cold IS the Cure! It is the cure for increased toxicity within the body which results in a depressed immune system (lowered resistance). Getting a cold is the body's way of "cleaning house", dumping toxins and exercising the immune system. Ever notice how good and healthy you feel after a bout with a cold or the flu.

Modern medicine focuses primarily on relieving uncomfortable symptoms, even though symptoms may be part of the healing process. For example, a fever increases the ability and effectiveness of the white blood cells in fighting illness. When a fever is reduced with drugs, the immune response is diminished and the illness is prolonged. Nearly eighty percent of infectious illnesses are viral and WILL NOT respond to antibiotics. The persistent use of antibiotics in our culture has shown to weaken the immune system and strengthen the virulence (power and nastiness) of bacteria. Many bacteria and infections have become resistant to even the most powerful antibiotics. The key to a speedy recovery for an infectious illness (whether it's viral or bacterial in origin) is to assist and support the body in the healing process.

Focus on cleansing the body and boosting the immune system.

- Drink plenty of unsweetened fluids. This is called a Flush. Herbal teas like Red Raspberry leaf, Catnip or Peppermint are great). My definition of "plenty of fluids" is to drink one full gallon (that's 128 ounces or 4-quarts) within a 24 hour period. Drink it hot or cold. Just drink it.
- Take immune stimulating herbs such as Immune Boost (see page 230) or Anti-Plague Formula (see page 219) every waking hour.
- Make sure your channels of elimination are working well. Use Colon Cleanse (see page 254) if you are not having 2-3 bowel movements daily. Do a Liver-Gallbladder Flush (page 257) or a Kidney-Bladder Flush (page 259) if necessary.
- Take SuperNutrition (see page 217) 2 to 3 times daily to boost your dietary nutritional supply .
- Drink fresh juices (carrot is best). Follow the dietary recommendations on page 243.
- Do the Cold Sheet Treatment below and review the Incurables Checklist (page 251) for additional "things to do".

Next time you feel a cold, flu or something even more serious coming on, rather than going for the drugs, work with the body and build your health. Take your herbs. Drink your teas and juice. Slow down and rest. Work with the body's natural healing processes rather than suppressing them. Remember, the body has an intelligence greater than all of medical science.

COLD SHEET TREATMENT

I know, this sounds like it may be a sorority or fraternity prank, but it is actually a very powerful healing technique. The purpose of the cold sheet treatment is to artificially induce or increase the body's temperature thereby accelerating the bodies immune response. The important thing to remember anytime heat is used with the body is to keep very well hydrated. A high temperature in a well hydrated body is safe and even healthy. The temperature can raise to 103 or 104 degrees Fahrenheit. However if the body is dehydrated and the temperature is raised, the body can overheat causing seizure or damage. Drinking plenty of fluids is more than sipping a savory tea. It is drinking until your stomach is full and then drinking some more. As follows, I will describe the cold sheet treatment as taught by Dr. John Christopher and then a few modifications that can be made.

Indications: The cold sheet treatment is used during the course of any infectious illness such as a cold or the flu. It can also be used with chronic degenerative illness.

Contraindications: Small children, the very elderly, heart disease or moderate to severe hypertensive (high blood pressure) conditions, extreme weakness and debility (are not recommended to do the Cold Sheet Treatment unless carefully supervised by a healthcare professional.) This procedure unmodified is quite rigorous so if you are inexperienced or if your patient is constitutionally very weak use your good judgment to modify the program.

This procedure is not to be done alone. Have one or two people administer this to the patient.

Supplies you will need:
1. Enema bag/set-up
2. Bulb syringe
3. Catnip tea
4. Yarrow or Red Raspberry tea
5. Powdered cayenne, ginger, and yellow mustard
6. 100% cotton sheet
7. Ice
8. Plastic/rubber sheet protector
9. Vaseline

The Cold Sheet Treatment

1. Begin with a cool enema of herbal tea (red raspberry or

catnip herbal tea is good). This is designed to cleanse and clear the bowel of loose fecal matter in preparation for step 2, the garlic injection. You may want to evacuate the bowel a couple of times. Each time hold the water in the bowel as long as you can before releasing. Be sure and lubricate the enema tip with oil or Vaseline.

2. Next use a rectal syringe from the drug store to introduce a garlic solution. In a blender mix 8-10 cloves of fresh garlic in 1 cup of water, and 1 cup of apple cider vinegar. For many this is the most intense part of this procedure. It is very safe, but does burn. Squirt in as much of the solution as you can. Keep the garlic solution in as long as you can, usually about 2 minutes before expelling. Even after expelling it, you will retain enough to do you good. The burning and cramping will subside in a couple of minutes.

3. Make a tea bag out of a sock and add into it one or more ounces of ginger root powder, yellow mustard powder and cayenne pepper powder. Fill the bath as hot as is tolerable without burning the skin. Before the patient gets in, it is important to coat the genitals with plenty of Vaseline. Put the patient in the bath and begin giving them hot/warm herbal tea to drink. Use yarrow (one of the best diaphoretics) or peppermint or ginger tea. The goal is to drink 6 to eight full cups of tea. It is the helpers job to get as much tea as possible into the patient. If the patient becomes faint or light-headed place a cold washcloth on the forehead. Cayenne tincture in the mouth will also prevent faintness. If the muscles become rigid or begin to spasm use lobelia tincture orally. Keep the patient in the tub for at least a half hour. Usually by 20 minutes they'll be aching to get out, but keep them in as long a possible drinking tea until 'it's coming out their ears'.

4. Prepare a double sized cotton sheet (it must be 100% cotton) by soaking it in a sink or tub of water and ice. Use lots of ice. Prepare the patients bed by putting a plastic sheet or lining against the mattress under the bed sheets. When the patient stands up out of the bath wrap the ice cold sheet around him/her. Then escort them to bed wrapped in the sheet. Tuck them into bed, sheet and all, then cover with

natural fiber blankets. Wrap them up in a cozy cocoon with a towel around the head leaving a face opening. Dr. Christopher recommends coating the soles of the feet with a garlic paste, then putting socks on the feet before putting them in bed. The paste is made by mixing mashed garlic with petroleum jelly. You can use the garlic that you strained from step two.

5. By lying in the sheet for several hours (preferably over night), the body will continue to sweat toxins out of the body. Often the sheet will be stained with these toxins. Keep the patient in bed for at least 2-3 hours.

6. Upon arising sponge off with apple cider vinegar and water (half and half) before taking a shower. This will wipe the toxins off the skin so they won't be reabsorbed during the shower.

7. Give the patient only fruit or vegetable juices and herbal teas for the next 1 to 3 days to provide a more thorough cleansing. Of course you should continue taking immune boosting herbs and herbal formula such as Echinacea, Goldenseal, Cats Claw, Immune Boost or Anti-Plague Formula.

There are countless modifications to this procedure. For example with a child, you can simply put them in warm bath, have them drink some herbal tea, give them immune boost, then tuck them into bed. However, for the full impact and benefit, follow the full procedure (don't wimp out on the enemas or the cold sheet because it sounds harsh or radical).

INCURABLE CHECKLIST

The incurables program as originally taught by Dr. John Christopher is designed to cleanse the body and assist the healing response. In my clinic, I have expanded on many of his ideas in order to cleanse the body and initiate healing. The key to healing is to work on cleansing and building all the systems of the body. Do everything and you will get well. As follows is a checklist of "things" that can be done to boost and re-build a healthier body. Of course you won't be able to do every single thing on the checklist every single day. Customize a program that will fit the patients needs. Healing the sick or injured body is rigorous work that takes some diligence. Put forth the effort and you will be rewarded.

1. **Juice/Herb Tea** = 1 gallon per day (This is inclusive of everything you drink during the day) Use to flush toxins and impurities from the body as well as nourish and stimulate the immune system.

2. **100% Vegetarian-Vegan Diet** - emphasize organic fruits and vegetables. If you are seriously ill consume only fresh carrot juice. Eight to sixteen ounces every waking hour (about a gallon of carrot juice daily). Do not eat solid foods if your condition is serious. Once you are off the juices you can go to a diet of fruits, vegetables, raw nuts and seeds, and soaked and sprouted beans and grains. Find organic produce grown locally. Absolutely no animal flesh, eggs, milk or milk products (cheese, yogurt, butter, etc.). No cooked foods (breads, baked potatoes, tofu, etc.)

3. Perform the **Cold Sheet Treatment** on a weekly basis, practice this once or twice with a friend so you will be confident using this powerful healing tool.

4. Consume no alcoholic beverages, caffeine, soda pop, or foods with artificial flavors, colors, etc.

5. SuperNutrition - 3 times per day (2 Tablespoons)

6. Immune Boost - (Echinacea combination) take every waking hour

7. Cayenne pepper - 1 teaspoon 3x/day or use capsules - work up to this dosage

8. Garlic - 8 to 10 cloves per day if really ill, 2 to 3 per day for maintenance

9. Wear only natural fiber clothing

10. No perfumes, lotions, chemicals worn on the body

11. No refined flours or sugars in the diet - only whole grains and starches

12. Carrot Juice - 8 cups daily - count this towards your 1 gallon per day

13. Freshly ground flaxseed 2-4 Tablespoons sprinkled over salad or food every day

14. Colon Cleanse page 222, to insure 2 to 3 normal bowel movements every day

15. Colon Detox, page 223 every third week
16. Liver Flush Program every other week
17. Liver-Gallbladder Formula - take during Liver flush
18. Drink Liver Detox Tea - 3 to 6 cups daily during Liver Flush
19. Kidney Flush Program alternate with Liver Flush Program
20. Drink Kidney-Bladder Tea - 3 to 6 cups daily during Kidney Flush
21. Kidney-Bladder Formula - take during Kidney Flush
22. Blood Cleansing Formula - Take 3 times daily
23. Essiac Tea - take 3 ounces morning and evening
24. Potassium Broth - 3 to 6 cups daily
25. Hot/Cold Hydrotherapy - focus on afflicted area 15 minutes 2 to 5x/daily
26. Dry skin brushing 2x/daily
27. Complete Tissue Repair ointment applied to afflicted area 3 to 6x/daily
28. Complete Tissue Repair syrup 1-3 teaspoons taken 3 times daily
29. Castor oil packs with hot water bottle 2-3x/daily over afflicted area
30. High Enemas 2-3x/week
31. Cold Sheet Treatment each week
32. Massage - daily w/olive oil - Foot Reflexology should be done as well
33. Exercise - for one hour each day - walking is best
34. Sun/Air bath 15 minutes daily - work up to this much time
35. Deep Breathing Exercises Daily
36. Barefoot on the grass 15 minutes daily
37. Take a short nap daily
38. Meditation - work up to 45 minutes daily - breath observation meditation and other meditation that you find appropriate in your studies.
39. Prayer 2 to 3 times daily
40. Think only uplifting positive thoughts
41. Help others

42. Discover your mission and purpose in life. Look to your illness/injury as a spiritual awaking. An opportunity for introspection and self-discovery.

43. Focus on Healing your life, not just your body.

44. Forgive and let go of past hurts, traumas, betrayals, etc. You can not heal if you do not release fear, anger, hate, guilt, etc. Hanging on to negative feelings will canker your soul. Repent (change your heart) and Forgive (let go of negativity). You can even forgive yourself—what a concept!

45. Read *Healing into Life and Death* by Stephen Levine. You must study, grasp and practice the principles that are taught in this book. Our life and our healing is more than just our body.

46. Become a student of your healing. Strive to learn from it.

47. Above all follow the inner voice of your spirit. It will guide, direct and teach you what you need to do. The road to health (spiritual and physical) is not designed to be easy, it will be a spiritual journey of discovering who you really are.

CLEANSING THE COLON

Cancer of the colon is the leading cancer, when men and women are combined. It is the leading cause of cancer deaths. Because of dietary changes over the last century, most of us have inherited a weak or sluggish bowel. When we add to that a poor diet that is low in fiber and nutrition and high in chemicals and toxins, the resulting constipation leads to the re-absorption of waste into the bloodstream. Diverticulosis, or bowel pockets, are a ballooning out of the intestinal tissue. When these become inflamed, diverticulosis may result. Bowel pockets, once thought to afflict only about 30% of the older population, are now estimated to affect nearly everyone both old and young alike. The appendix can become impacted with fecal material and become inflamed resulting in appendicitis. Once thought to be a useless organ, now we understand that the appendix actually has a function with our immune system as well as acting as a lubricant for the rest of the large intestines. An oil can for the colon (large intestines) if you will.

When toxic waste matter is left to stagnate in the lower bowel tract, the system becomes polluted with poisonous gases which congest and irritate the surrounding organs, causing adhesions, and other ailments, such as chronic constipation, diverticulosis, appendicitis, irritable bowel syndrome, leg ulcers, headaches, allergies, etc. In fact, a congested and constipated colon will hinder the elimination of toxins from your body. Most people have pounds of fecal matter that is stored in the colon which is toxifying the system and keeping food from being assimilated (absorbed). It is not hard to understand that cells can become weakened and even cancerous if constantly exposed to a toxic, unfriendly environment. Because of this sluggish and slowly responsive condition, most people eat far more than their bodies actually require in an effort to feel satisfied. The body cries for nourishment with pangs of hunger, only to be fed nutritionally deficient foods. People eat and eat and are not satisfied because of lack of good nourishment. This is why SuperNutrition (see page 217) is a valuable supplement. It satisfies the body's nutritional cries. After the bowel is cleansed, food is better absorbed and assimilated and many find they require far less food. Often only half of what they were accustomed to and they enjoy a tremendous increase in energy.

The body is designed to gain the nutritional value from foods through the cellular structures of the small and large intestines, instead of being trapped in a maze of wastage, and inhibited by the hard fecal castings on the intestinal walls. When the body is completely clean, herbal aids will no longer be necessary.

A good lower bowel or colon remedy should be designed to heal, build and strengthen the colon. Many herbal products are simply strong laxatives and do not build and strengthen. As your body begins to heal and become healthier, you should require less and less of the herbs to assist your bowels in normal function. It makes sense that if you are taking something that is building health, that as time passes, you will require less. Alternately, something that stimulates the body into a certain function will require more and more because the body continues to deteriorate rather than get healthier. Don't get caught into that trap. It is safe to assume you are not correcting the problem, but covering up the symptom. Strong herbal or over-the-counter laxatives liquefy the fecal matter, which allows for toxins to be more easily absorbed and are not recommended.

COLON CLEANSE PROGRAM

Colon Cleanse

This formula is used to cleanse, heal and strengthen the entire digestive tract. Colon Cleanse stimulates the peristaltic action (the intestinal muscular movement) of the colon and over time strengthens the muscles of the large intestines. Colon Cleanse helps to disinfect, soothe and heal the mucous membranes lining the entire digestive system. Colon Cleanse aids in digestion, relieves gas, cramps and cleanses the gallbladder and bile ducts, destroying candida albicans overgrowth and parasites, promoting a healthy intestinal flora.

Begin the use of Colon Cleanse with 1 capsule during or following the evening meal (some prefer breakfast). This formula works best when taken with food. The following morning you should notice an increase in your bowel action and in the amount of fecal matter that you eliminate. The consistency should also be softer. If there is not a noticeable change in bowel behavior, increase the dosage by one capsule each night until a noticeable change occurs. A bowel movement corresponding with each meal (2 to 3 per day) is considered healthy bowel function.

With Colon Cleanse, the lower bowel tonic, we feed and nourish the eliminative organs and allow the colon to work on its own. **Aloe Vera** powder is used because of its ability to cause contractions of the bowel wall muscles. It contains a phytochemical (phyto means herb) that will cause any smooth or intestinal muscle to move. **Senna** and **Cascara sagrada** are also used because of their mild laxative and tonifying and strengthening effect on the muscles of the intestines. **Barberry** is a great liver herb which will help the body in the detoxification of toxins that may be stirred up in the cleansing process. **Ginger** and **Fennel** help with digestion and gas build up. **Garlic** is antibacterial and anti-fungal, helping to eliminate harmful organisms while promoting the re-establishment of healthy intestinal flora. **Cayenne pepper** is used because it acts to stop any intestinal bleeding, ulceration or irritation. While cayenne may seem to be a strong stimulating herb, it is actually very soothing on the digestive tract. In fact, cayenne pepper is used to treat stomach or duodenal ulcers. **Black Walnut, Clove** and **Wormwood** are used in this formula because they have the ability to kill and expel parasites as they might infect the digestive tract.

Colon Detox

This formula is used to cleanse, purify and detoxify the colon, bowels and intestines. Colon Detox soothes and strengthens the entire intestinal tract. Colon Detox is a strong purifier and intestinal vacuum, helping to draw out old fecal matter from the walls of the colon and from any bowel pockets. Colon Detox is uniquely formulated to soften old fecal matter for easy elimination. It aids in the removal of poisons, toxins, parasites and heavy metals. It is also used as a remedy for intestinal inflammation such as diverticulitis, colitis or irritable bowel syndrome. This product is also used effectively for diarrhea or food poisoning.

Colon Detox can be used in powder or capsule form. For an intensive colon cleansing (recommended 2 to 4 times yearly, depending on your diet), take Colon Detox as directed - 1 heaping teaspoon or 12 capsules, 5 times daily. It is important to take with plenty of water and increase your Colon Cleanse capsules by one to assure 2 to 3 normal bowel movements per day. Taken without sufficient water Colon Detox can be constipating. Follow this regimen for five or six days.

Colon Detox contains the following herbs: **Apple pectin**, **Bentonite clay** and **charcoal** all have the ability to pull up to forty times their weight in toxins from the walls and pockets in the colon. If you have ever experienced a clay mask and felt the strong astringent pulling, imagine having a clay mask on the inside pulling toxins out. **Flax seed** will soothe and soften old hardened fecal matter allowing for easier elimination and **Psyllium** seeds and husks act as bulking agents to move things along. Finally **Fennel** is one of the greatest herbs to reduce gas or flatulence. This simple and effective product has helped many.

LIVER-GALLBLADDER FLUSH PROGRAM

The liver is responsible for handling most of our energy needs. It takes raw material from foods and breaks them down into their basic components. It creates and stores sugars for both immediate and long-term energy use. If the liver is congested or diseased it will not receive or send out enough blood sugar and your energy will drop. If you're experiencing chronic lack of energy, especially after meals, focus on cleansing the liver.

The liver is also vital in detoxifying and neutralizing toxins within the body, particularly as it is absorbed from the digestive tract. Because our environment is full of stressful chemicals, such as food additives, preservatives, pesticides, herbicides, etc., it is vital that we have a healthy functioning liver.

A periodic Liver Flush, in addition to a healthy lifestyle can greatly benefit overall health.

We strongly recommend doing the Colon Cleanse Program before beginning the liver flush. As the name implies, a flush will wash and cleanse the tissues of the body, so expect that you'll make frequent trips to the bathroom. The herbs in this cleansing program not only help to eliminate waste and toxins from the liver and gallbladder but also help to build and strengthen these organs to help them function more efficiently.

This is a one week program designed to flush, cleanse and strengthen the liver and gallbladder. The program consists of 3 parts, the morning drink, the tea and the herbal extract.

A. Begin each morning with the following drink:
   In a blender mix the following:
   1. 8 ounces of organic orange, apple or grape juice.
   2. 8 ounces of distilled water
   3. 1 to 4 cloves of fresh garlic
   4. 1 to 4 Tablespoons of organic extra virgin olive oil.
   5. 1 small (1/4 to 1") piece of fresh ginger root.

B. Make six to eight cups of the Liver detox tea. You may sweeten with pure maple syrup or honey. Drink all of this tea each day. Use 3 Tbs. of tea to make 8 cups.

C. Use the Liver-Gallbladder Formula 2 to 4 dropperfuls 3 or 4 times during the day. You may add this tincture to your tea as you drink it.

You should be eating a diet consisting of predominately fruits, vegetables and whole grains. Avoid meats, dairy, refined flour, sugars, salt (other than natural sea salt), coffee, any form of caffeine, anything carbonated, etc. During this week of liver cleansing, a castor oil fomentation should be used over the liver three times on non-consecutive days. Use a sauna or steam room to promote sweating. Follow this program for 7 to 10 consecutive days.

KIDNEY
Bladder Flush Program

The kidneys are another important elimination channel. Many nitrogen containing wastes products, such as ammonia and urea are excreted in the urine. The liver transforms any fat-soluble toxins into water soluble compounds that can then be eliminated through the kidneys. This Kidney-Bladder Flush is disinfecting and is very useful for urinary tract infections, often working within a day or two when strong drugs have failed.

It is very important that the bowels have been cleansed and are moving before you begin a flush. We recommend following the Colon Cleansing Program prior to either the Kidney or the Liver Flush. Use enough Colon Cleanse Formula while doing either flush so that you are having 2 to 3 normal bowel movements per day. As the name implies, a flush will wash and cleanse the tissues of the body, so expect that you'll make frequent trips to the bathroom. The herbs in this and all of the other cleansing programs not only help to eliminate waste and toxins from the body but also help to build and strengthen the individual organs to help them function more efficiently.

We recommend this flush every three to four months or as needed. Whether you have a kidney condition or not, this kidney cleansing routine will be beneficial. Of course, if you have edema (swelling), stones, recurrent urinary tract infections or any kidney/bladder concerns this program is a must.

Kidney Flush Program

A. Begin each morning with the following drink:
   In a blender mix the following:

   1. Juice of one lemon and one lime

   2. 16 to 32 ounces of distilled water

   3. A pinch of cayenne pepper (this is the best circulation enhancing herb)

   4. Optional - pure maple syrup (just a little) to taste

B. Make six to eight cups of the Kidney/Bladder Tea. You may sweeten it with pure maple syrup or honey. Drink all of this tea each day. Use 3 Tbs. of tea to make 8 cups.

C. Use the Kidney/Bladder Formula 2 to 4 dropperfuls 3 or 4 times during the day. You may add this tincture to your tea as you drink it.

You should be eating a diet consisting of predominately fruits, vegetables and whole grains. Avoid meats, dairy, refined flour, sugars, salt (other than natural sea salt), coffee, any form of caffeine, anything carbonated, etc. Sauna or steam room use is encouraged to promote sweating and cleansing the skin and pores. Follow this program for 7 to 10 consecutive days.

HEALING SOFT TISSUE INJURIES

There are 3 essential keys for healing any type of injury. These are circulation, nutrition and elimination. When the body is injured, whether the result of an accident (acute trauma), or through repeated stress (cumulative trauma), the body responds with inflammation, swelling, muscle spasm and pain. As a result, the area of injury becomes congested resulting in poor circulation. Good blood flow or circulation is essential to healing. As we know, blood carries the healing nutrients we take into the cells of our bodies and carries away the wastes from injury or normal metabolism to be eliminated from the body. The blood must be nutrient rich and the circulation must be good to carry away the waste in order for proper and timely healing to occur. Here are some suggestions on how you can help your body heal more quickly.

ICE or Cryotherapy: Injury to the body often results in inflammation, pain and muscles spasms. The initial course of action should be to calm the inflammation by putting ice on the injury. Always begin your treatment of an acute injury with ice. As a general rule ice for 10 to 20 minutes every waking hour for the first 24 to 72 hours depending on the severity of the injury. Icing longer than 20 minutes at a time, especially with direct ice contact (i.e. Your foot in a bucket of ice water) can be counterproductive (the body increases the circulation to the area as a defense against frostbite). Soft gel ice packs can be purchased or you can make your own with ice cubes in a zip lock bag. Frozen un-popped popcorn kernels in a zip-lock work quite well and hold the cold for a long time.

Hot & Cold Hydrotherapy: This is one of the most powerful healing modalities. More powerful than drugs, herbs or even massage. The cold will drive the blood from the painful area, and the heat will bring the nutrient rich blood back to the area. By alternating hot and cold, you can literally force the blood in and out of the area, thereby delivering more nutrients and carrying away more waste and inflammation, greatly speeding up the healing.

Directions: Using water directly against the skin is by far the most effective way to speed up healing. In the shower or using a hand held shower wand, run the water over the afflicted area as hot as you can stand it for 30 to 60 seconds. Then turn the water all the way to cold for 30 to 60 seconds. (It's okay to hoot and holler). Lighten up the intensity for Children, the elderly, and those who are constitutionally very weak. (If your health is a question, you are allowed to use your common sense). Alternate back and forth with the hot and cold for 15 minutes. Do this 7 to 10 times per day. The shower experience can be intense and not everyone is willing to do this. Next best, but not nearly as effective, is to alternate ice pack and heating pad. Five to eight minutes of heat, followed by five to eight minutes of ice. Alternate for 30 minutes. Do this 7 to 10 times per day. Can't do this 7 times per day? Do your best. Anything is better than nothing.

Deep Heating Oil or ointment (see page 226) is a marvelous healing ointment that can be rubbed directly into the painful area (provided it is not an open wound). It is a POWERFUL deep penetrating heating ointment that relieves pain, inflammation, spasm and stiffness in joints, tendons, ligaments and muscle. It will also increase the cellular repair and greatly reduce healing time. Use this oil for arthritis, bursitis, tendonitis, carpal tunnel, sprains, strains, and any muscle or bone pain. To intensify the treatment rub the ointment into the body each time after a very hot shower or the hot and cold hydrotherapy.

Complete Tissue Repair Syrup and Ointment (see page 224)

This amazing formula greatly accelerates the repair of both soft tissue injuries (sprains and strains) as well as hard tissue injuries (fractures). CTR ointment can be used externally where there may be cuts or abrasions that the deep heat oil will make uncomfortable. Syrup should be taken 1 to 3 teaspoons three times daily. Comfrey leaf or root tea may be used in place of the syrup. Three to six cups daily.

Castor Oil Packs - (see page 211 for instructions). This venerable form of treatment is tried and true. Whether used to clear out a congested liver or pull the inflammation out of a chronic injury, a castor oil pack can be very healing and an effective way to speed the healing of injured tissues.

MASSAGE THERAPY

Massage is one the earliest and still one of the most effective therapy modalities. It is easy to do, requires little training, just a willing heart and hands. Of course, when it comes to massage, nothing quite compares to a well trained, experienced, gifted massage therapist. Space does not permit a detailed discussion on how to massage. There are many excellent books and videos available. Take the time and learn the basics.

Physiologic Effects of Massage:

1. Increases blood flow
2. Increases lymph and venous drainage
3. Increases heart rate
4. Increase blood pressure
5. Decreases edema or swelling
6. Stretches and/or breaks adhesions (scar tissue)
7. Increases urine production
8. Increases respiration
9. Sedates motor and sensory nerve activity
10. Removes lactic acid from musculature
11. Increases peristalsis if done over abdomen
12. Decreases muscle spasm

Indications: pain and muscle spasm, subacute or chronic conditions to the soft tissue; subacute and healing fractures; sprains; strains; bursitis; tendonitis; muscle contraction/tension headache; arthritis; stiff joints; bruises; and pain that radiates.

Contraindications (don't do it); Skin infections or open cuts and abrasions; Inflammation with pus; Burns (including sunburns); skin rashes or infections; malignancies (unless you know what you are doing and why you are doing it).

ENERGY AND HEALING

Therapeutic touch can be a very important part in the treatment and management of illness and injury. There are many systems that use "energy" and touch as a healing modality. CranioSacral Therapy and Reiki both use "energetic methods" in healing and relieving pain. One method described by Dr. John Upledger, the founder and developer of CranioSacral Therapy is the Direction of Energy Technique. He describes it as follows:

"Basically, the "direction of energy" technique is a very simple one. Place one hand (hand 1) on the opposite side of the body part from the bruise, cut, boil, abscess, sprain, strain, infection or bump. Point the fingers of this hand at the problem so that they direct energy at it. These fingers (1, 2, or 3 of them) will usually be at approximately right angles to the skin surface which they are touching. Now make a cup of your other hand (hand 2) over the problem so that your hand edges are touching around the problem but not directly on it. Imagine a force traveling from hand 1 to hand 2. The injured area will begin to pulsate as the energy travels from one hand to the other. After a few minutes the pulsation's will diminish and the area will soften and start to feel better. The process is repeated two or three times daily until the symptoms feel better and the involved tissue looks better. We think of this process as sending reinforcements that strengthen natural body defenses and healing processes." (*Your Inner Physician and You*, page 144, 1991).

TWIN TENNIS BALLS IN TANDEM
or "Still Point Inducer"

Our skulls are comprised of 22 different bones which interlock with each other much like folding our hands together interlacing the fingers. These bones do not fuse together like a coconut as we get older but actively move with a subtle expansion and contraction. This cranial respiratory motion or rhythm is independent of the rhythms of our heart beat or breathing. One of the purposes of this cranial bone movement is to pump or circulate the cerebrospinal fluid or CFS. It is vital to our health that the cranial bones are able to move in their prescribed rate and rhythm (about 6 to 12 cycles per minute). A good "shotgun" technique for enhancing the normal motion of these cranial bones can be done by lying with tennis balls under the back of your head to create what is referred to as a "Still Point". This wonderful technique was first taught and described by Dr. John Upledger in his book CranioSacral Therapy. The momentary stopping of the CranioSacral rhythm (a "still point") is like pushing a reset button triggering the CranioSacral system's self-correcting abilities, which in turn can have profound beneficial effects throughout the body.

This technique can relax the connective tissues (muscles, etc.) throughout the body, and restore normal nervous system responses as it relates to stress. It is beneficial for acute and chronic musculoskeletal lesions, including degenerative arthritis. It can lower fever as much as four degrees Fahrenheit. It can reduce cerebral or pulmonary congestion, and edema or swelling. It has been used to improve auto-immune diseases, autistic behavior of children, and anxiety.

This technique can benefit most individuals to some degree and is rarely, if ever, harmful.

In addition, the tennis balls can be used all up and down the spine to relieve aches and pains massaging out trigger points. Even a single tennis ball, pressed between the wall and tight spots on your back, rolling back and forth can effectively massage and soothe tight muscles.

This technique should not be used during the acute stages of stroke or head injury.

How to get started: Two tennis balls (or racquetballs) are put together next to each other (in tandem) so that they are touching one another. This can be done most easily by putting them together in the toe of a sock and tying the sock in a knot to hold the balls firmly together.

Instructions: Recline on your back, on the floor, bed or couch and place the tennis balls under your head so that the entire weight of your head rests on the two tennis balls. They are placed about 1/3 the way "up" the back of the head rather than in the crook of the neck or on the muscles. The level of the tennis balls is slightly above the openings of the ears on the back of the head.

Allow the weight of your head to rest upon the tennis balls for 10 -15 minutes. Relax comfortably. You may shift your position slightly in order to maintain symmetry and comfort, but do so gently and gradually.

Repeat this daily. A good practice is to keep the tennis balls by your bed and use when you first lie down at night.

WALKING

Walking is the easiest program to start. No special skill is required - you already know how to walk - and it's always ready when you are. You don't have to worry about gathering up exercise gear, getting out equipment, or driving to a gym. All you have to do is walk out your front door. In case of bad weather, go to a shopping mall or a gym and walk on a treadmill. They have become very popular for early morning walkers.

While many fitness buffs may look down on walking as being tame compared to running or more competitive sports, experts show that in getting and staying fit and free from injury walking is the best. You can obtain maximum fitness from walking alone; However, as with all exercise it only works if you do. The key is consistency. Day in and day out. The key of course is developing a routine.

We recommend a good pair of walking or running shoes with a good cushioning in the insole. While not essential, they will support and feel better on your feet. Walking up hills or walking at a quick pace will build cardio-vascular fitness. Walking alone allows you to be with your thoughts and nature, while walking with a friend you can enjoy conversation. Many enjoy walking with a cassette player listening to lively music or books-on-tape or foreign language lessons. Your walking time need not be filled with boredom.

Plan your walk each day. I find that if I make an appointment with myself, I am more likely to keep it than if I don't. Another secret is to share your goal to walk with someone else. You should finish your walk feeling like you could have done more. It is not recommended to walk or exercise to the point of fatigue or exhaustion.

Begin with this Eight Week Program

Week One: Walk 10 minutes each day - Walk at least 5 or 6 days during the week

Week Two: Increase to 15 minutes per day

Week Three: 20 minutes per day

Week Four: 25 minutes per day

Week Five: 30 minutes per day

Week Six: 35 minutes per day

Week Seven: 40 minutes per day

Week Eight: 45 minutes per day

Having built a base of conditioning, you should continue to walk 45 minutes or more per day. Plan walks at the mountains and trails. Walking is a great way to experience nature.

BREATH OBSERVATION MEDITATION

Many shy away from things like yoga and meditation fearing that it is some form of Eastern "non-christian" religious practice. Put in western terms these are nothing more than stretching and relaxing exercises and do not need to have ties to any religion or philosophy. When we practice any form of relaxation, bio-feedback or meditation, we can learn better to relax, reduce pain or stress, break out of old habits and patterns, and free the mind to allow you to reach your potential.

In a time when our minds are filled with distractions, and so many diversions vying for our attention, it is important that we learn to calm and clear the mind. By following the practice of breath observation we can become more "mindful" and free ourselves from becoming so easily distracted from the things that really matter most in life.

To use your breathing to nurture mindfulness, just tune in to the feeling of it. . . the feeling of the breath coming into your body and the feeling of the breath leaving your body. That's all. Just feeling the breath. Breathing and knowing your breathing. This doesn't mean deep breathing or forcing your breathing, or trying to feel something special, or wondering whether you're doing it right. It doesn't mean thinking about your breathing, either. It's just a bare bones awareness of the breath moving in and the breath moving out.

It doesn't have to be for a long time at any one stretch. Using the breath to bring us back to the present moment takes no time at all, only a shift in attention. But great adventures await you if you give yourself a little time to string moments of awareness together, breath by breath, moment to moment.

TRY: Starting with one full in-breath as it come in, one full out-breath as it goes out, keeping your mind open and free for just this moment, just this breath. Abandon all ideas of getting somewhere or having anything happen. Just keep returning to the breath when the mind wanders, stringing moments of mindfulness together, breath by breath.

Begin with Breath Observation Meditation by sitting in a comfortable position with your back straight and your eyes lightly closed. Loosen any tight clothing. Focus your attention on your breathing, and follow the contours of the cycle through inhalation and exhalation, noting, if you can, the points at which one phase changes into the other.

Do this for five minutes once a day. Your goal is simply to keep your attention on the breath cycle and observe. It may speed up or slow down; it may get deeper or more shallow; it may seem to stop for a time. Whatever happens with your breathing, innocently observe it, without anticipating or resisting any changes.

You will find that at times your attention drifts away from your breath and goes to a thought in the mind, some sensation in the body, a sound in the environment or some emotional feeling. Whenever you notice that you are not observing the breath, gently bring your attention back to your breathing.

There is no failure in a meditative experience. Dr. Deepak Chopra explains that when you meditate you will experience one of three things.

First: you may feel bored or restless and your mind may become filled with random thoughts or worries. This is an indication that deep-rooted stresses and emotions are being released from your system. By continuing with meditation, you will allow these impurities to be removed from your mind and body.

Second: You may fall asleep. If you fall asleep in mediation, it is an indication that you need more rest during other times of the day.

Third: you may slip into the gap. When your breath becomes very settled and refined, you can slip into the gap between your thoughts, beyond sound, and beyond breath.

Recommended Reading: *Wherever You Go, There You Are,* by Jon Kabat-Zinn

Rules for Getting Well

1. Learn to accept whatever decision is made. Do your best to keep your peace of mind. Peace is a healer.

2. Let the other person make a mistake and learn. This is so much better than standing over people and supervising every move. Learn to give others the opportunity to grow and grow up. We are bound to make mistakes. Let's not gloat over them and live in remorse about them.

3. Learn to forgive and get on with your life. Many studies have shown that forgiving enhances health and helps prevent chemical changes in the body that may lead to disease.

4. Be thankful and bless people. These are two of the main secrets to a healthy life.

5. Live in harmony.

6. Don't talk about your misfortunes or illnesses. It doesn't do any good for you or the person you tell, and it presents an opportunity for them to do the same to you. Save it for your doctor. He's paid to listen to your troubles.

7. Don't gossip. Gossip that comes through the grapevine is usually sour grapes. Be the person who speaks and stands up for the one not present.

8. Spend 10 minutes a day meditating on how you can become a better person. Replace negative thoughts with positive ones.

9. Exercise daily. Keep your spine and joints limber, develop your abdominal muscles, expand your lungs with specific exercises on a regular schedule.

10. Walk 10 minutes barefoot in the dewy grass or sand every day. You'll sleep better.

11. No smoking or drinking alcohol. Both nicotine and alcohol are depressant drugs. Both require energy to detoxify the body, which energy is better used for life healing processes.

12. Go to bed by 9 p.m. when you can. If you are tired during the day, rest more. Rest allows the body to give its full attention and energy to healing and rebuilding tissues. Write down your problems at the end of the day and go over them first thing in the morning when you are refreshed, so you can look at them with a fresh mind and body.

YOGA STRETCHES

The key to a healthy spine is strength and flexibility. People who practice yoga regularly are reported to have less lower back or neck pain that any other group studied. Begin with a video or join a class, but get started. Ideally you can find a class or instructor who can work with you and your needs and ability. Be gentle and patient with your progress. Yoga is not competative.

SEA SALT

Throw away your table salt and begin using salt balanced with nature's full spectrum of minerals. This salt has been known to lower high blood pressure and improve health. Remember natural sea salt that has not been super heated and refined is a nutritious supplement to your diet and is beneficial to health. One reason so many people use excessive amounts of refined salt on their food is because their bodies are craving all of the nutrients that are naturally found in salt (the potassium, magnesium, calcium, silicon, zinc, iron, copper, plus 80+ trace minerals, in addition to sodium and chloride). When the body craves salt and you give it only refined sodium and chloride (with a little added iodine) then the body is not satisfied and will continue to crave natural salt. If you salt your food before you taste it, or crave salt, please, please, please begin using a sea salt that contains all of the minerals you need, not just sodium, chloride and a little iodine.

WATER

Drinking water is one of the major sources of environmental toxins that can harm your body. Fortunately, it is one that you can do something about.

Here are some suggestions:

- Never drink water that tastes like chlorine, even if it means going thirsty. Order bottled water if you are eating out.
- Avoid using tap water for drinking or cooking. It is unfit for human consumption, because impurities from plumbing and the insides of hot-water tanks more readily leach out through it.
- Use bottled water only as a temporary solution. It is much too expensive for regular use, and often bottled water is tap water in disguise. Home purifying systems are a good investment. Don't rely on tests provided by the sales company. We recommend distilled or reverse osmosis water for drinking and cooking. Distilled or reverse osmosis water is best for making herbal teas because the water is "empty". Unlike mineral water, distilled water has the ability to draw out the phytochemicals (the herbal properties) better than water that is already full of minerals. Contrary to what you may have heard, drinking distilled water will not leach the minerals out of your body, damaging your health.
- If finances prohibit you from buying bottled water or purchasing a filter, then you can at least allow the chlorine to evaporate off your drinking water by setting it out in a pitcher for two to three hours before you drink or use it. Set out several pitchers of water each night for your drinking and cooking needs.

Purchase a filter for your shower head. It will remove the chlorine and make the air fit for breathing and washing while taking a shower. You can absorb more chlorine during a 20 minute shower than you can by drinking 8 glasses of chlorinated water.

- Surprisingly, a major cause of health problems today stem from dehydration. Inadequate daily intake of water has been indicated in many conditions ranging from constipation and asthma to stomach ulcers and chronic inflammatory diseases. Often strong medications are used to control symptoms when drinking water will heal the body and cure the problem. By simply increasing your water intake you can greatly improve your health. A 150 pound person should drink a minimum of 64 oz. per day (that's 1/2 gallon). Adjust the amount according to your weight, add roughly one eight ounce glass for every 25 pounds over 150 pounds you weigh, and add one glass of water for every 25 pounds overweight you are.

Drink your water. You will be astounded at how it will improve your health. At first you will need to urinate more frequently, but as your body adapts to drinking more water your body will adjust and you won't be running to the bathroom quite so often.

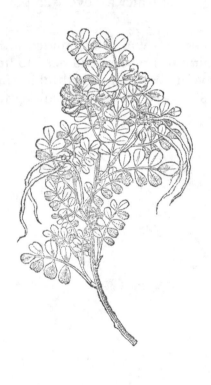

Chapter 20

GROWING YOUR OWN MEDICINES

Why a section on gardening in a first aid manual?! Because it's important. It really is. The best supply to have on hand is one that is ever present and that you've become familiar with. Develop a relationship with your herbs. Get to know them and some day they may repay the friendship. I encourage everyone to begin planting in their yards, in planter boxes or pots, herbs that can be used medicinally. Many of these herbs once planted will grow and maintain themselves. So if you are in no way shape or form going to put on the overalls and boots and head out to the back forty to dig in the dirt, plan on investing in a pound of each of the essential medicinal herbs to keep on hand. If you tincture them, they can last a life time. The message here is prepare. If you are prepared, you need not fear.

Many herbs are easy to grow and will flourish even in poor soil if they get enough sunshine and water. Most herbs necessary for first aid purposes grow well in temperate climates.

BUYING PLANTS: Some herbs grow very slowly. Consider getting an established plant from a friend or a nursery. Buy plants in the spring when the danger of frost is past and nurseries still have stocks of young, healthy plants.

Look for strong, healthy specimens with plenty of new growth and space in the pot. Avoid straggling, yellowing herbs in weed-choked pots or plants with roots emerging from the base. Loose soil implies recent replanting.

Examine the undersides of leaves for pests such as aphids, red spider mites, and whitefly. Try to check that plants are correctly labeled - mistakes can and do happen.

GROWING PLANTS

From Seed: It is best to sow annual and biennial herbs directly where they are intended to grow, following the packet instructions. Celery, chamomile, dill, and pot marigold are easy to grow. Perennials that grow well from seed include elecampane, fennel, Feverfew, hyssop, sage, wood Betony, catnip, thyme, St. John's wort, plantain, and skullcap. Dandelion and chickweed grow as weeds.

By Root Division: Divide roots with a small fork or sharp spade in early spring. Replant immediately and water thoroughly. Roman chamomile, peppermint and spearmint can be propagated by cutting and replanting the small offsets and runners.

From Cuttings: Woody perennial herbs are best propagated by cuttings taken from side shoots in late summer or early autumn. Set in water or plant directly in a pot keeping well watered. Try elder, hyssop, thyme, lavender, rosemary, and sage.

WHEN TO HARVEST

Choose a dry day and gather herbs once the morning dew has evaporated. The leaves of evergreens, such as hyssop and rosemary, can be collected anytime except on frosty days. Herbs can also be harvested whenever there is an immediate need.

Early Spring: Harvest roots such as dandelion.

Late Spring: Flowers; such as elder

Early to Midsummer: Flowers and flowering tops: chamomile, pot marigold, St. John's wort.

Aerial parts/leaves before flowering: catnip, dandelion, lemon balm, raspberry leaf, peppermint, plantain.

Mid to Late Summer: Aerial parts while flowering: boneset, chickweed, comfrey, marshmallow, Meadowsweet, peppermint, skullcap, thyme, blue vervain, yarrow.

Flowers: hops, lavender.

Leaves: Ginkgo.

Autumn: Roots/bulbs when the leaves have wilted: burdock (first year), echinacea, elecampane (2-3 year old roots), garlic, marshmallow, valerian, yellow dock, fennel.

Seeds or fruit when ripe: celery, chaste tree, dill elder, evening primrose.

ALOE VERA *(Aloe vera)*

Every home should have one or two aloe vera plants. This cactus requires little water, little light and will prove to be a valuable ally with burns and injuries.

Key Actions: cooling, soothing, a cell proliferant . Use for burns, cuts, abrasions.

Cultivation: This cactus requires a warm climate without excessive cold or freezing. Everyone should grow this as a house plant. Propagate from root divisions. Requires little water.

Harvest & Storage: It is recommended to use fresh. With a cut or a burn, fillet a leaf and apply the slab of aloe vera directly to the wound. Wrap to secure. Expect miracles. Can be stored, once peeled, ground up and preserved with a little vitamin C (ascorbic acid) powder. Keep refrigerated for up to 2 weeks.

CATNIP *(Nepeta cataria)*

Part of the mint family. "If you sow it cats won't know it, if you set it cats will get it". Yes cats love catnip. But if planted from the seed and left undisturbed cats will leave it alone. They are attracted to the oil from a broken or disturbed leaf. Lions, tigers, and leopards are not immune from the seductive lure of catnip.

Key Actions: Sedative, carminative. For headaches, upset stomachs.

Cultivation: Easily propagated from seeds or root divisions. Sow directly in your garden. Catnip thrives in a variety of soils from poor and dry to rich deep, and shaded. Plants will become more fragrant when grown in sandy soil in full sun.

Harvesting & Storage: Harvest the flowering tops. Dry the leaves and flowers in open air. Once dried the leaves crack from the stem easily and can be stored in plastic bags or a sealed jar.

CAYENNE *(Capsicum annuum)*

There are about 20 species and hundreds of varieties of Capsicum. I recommend habanero peppers as these are the hottest and will give you the most "bang for your buck".

Key Action: Stimulates blood circulation, aids digestion, relieves gas and colic.

Cultivation: Can be grown from seeds sown indoors 6-8 weeks before transplanting. Grow in full sun in rich sandy loam soil. A light soil will produce more than heavy clay soils.

Harvest & Storage: Harvest the ripened red (cayenne) or orange (habanero) fruit and string them up to dry. Be careful not to break the stem at the top of the fruit, which will cause it to spoil before drying. Peppers may take several weeks to dry.

CHAMOMILE *(Matricaria recutita & Chamaemelum nobile)*

Key Actions: Sedative, carminative (soothes stomach/ helps digestion), anti-inflammatory, antibacterial & antiseptic, bitter & prevents vomiting.

Cultivation: Prefers well-drained slightly acidic, moist or dry soil in full sun. Sow seeds in spring or autumn. Both single- and double-flowered varieties can be used medicinally.

Harvesting & Storage: Collect the flowers when they first open and use fresh or dry on trays. Store in a cool dry place. The flowers soon deteriorate with drying, and freezing can be better for long-term storage.

COMFREY *(Symphytum officinal)*

Also known at "boneknit" comfrey is one of the great healers of injury. Falsely accused of being harmful to the liver, comfrey now has a clean record and today there is no single man, women or child in any country who has been recorded as suffering toxic effects from taking comfrey leaf or root as medicine.

Key Action: cell proliferant speeding the growth and repair of damaged tissue due to illness or injury.

Cultivation: Comfrey is best propagated by dividing the roots in the spring or fall. A little piece of root will produce a plant. Once planted comfrey will be there forever. Comfrey will grow in almost any soil, but produces larger roots and more leaf material in a rich, deep, moist soil, high in organic matter and compost.

Harvesting & Storage: Harvest the leaves as the flowers bud up. You can harvest comfrey up to seven times per year. Dry comfrey leaf in the shade as leaves dried in the sun will quickly turn black.

DANDELION *(Taraxacum official)*

While your neighbors are trying to eradicate their dandelions, you can harvest yours for both medicinal and culinary purposes.

Key Actions: strengthen liver, gallbladder and kidney functions. Improves digestion. Anti-inflammatory. Increases bile secretions.

Cultivation: It is unlikely you will need to plant dandelion. However, you can harvest the seeds (remember how you used to blow them from the dried flower). Dandelion will grow in most soils, but will produce larger roots in a rich, deep, moist soil, well supplied with compost and well-rotted manure.

Harvesting & Storage: The root is harvested in autumn as the vegetative growth fades. The timing of the harvest affects the quality of the root. Roots harvested in summer (June - August) are less potent than roots harvested in September - October. Harvest leaves when they are still tender and sweet.

ECHINACEA *(Echinacea angustifolia, E. purpurea)*

Probably the most popular of Native American herbs. This powerful immune booster has a beautiful flower that should ornament every home.

Key Action: Immune stimulation, anti-inflammatory, accelerates wound healing.

Cultivation: Seeds can be difficult to germinate. Out of 100 seeds of E. angustifolia, I was only successful with 4. Purchasing an established plant or splitting a root stock is probably the best and easiest way to establish this hardy plant. Most echinacea grows in poor, rocky, slightly acidic to alkaline well-drained soils. Full sun is required. Keep well weeded, Echinacea doesn't like the competition.

Harvesting & Storage: Harvest the roots in autumn after the plants have gone to seed. Dry in shade or under forced heat (a dehydrator). Roots over one-inch in diameter can be split before drying.

GARLIC *(Allium sativum)*

Garlic is the most popular and pungent herb throughout the world. Used by virtually every culture past and present. Garlic is king of herbs and if limited to only one medicinal herb, garlic would be a worthy choice.

Key Actions: Endless culinary uses. Anti-bacterial, anti-fungal, antiviral, lowers high blood pressure, thins blood, lowers cholesterol.

Cultivation: Grow from nursery sets (bulbels), or by planting individual cloves. The outer cloves will produce superior plants. A moist sandy soil moderately rich in humus with full sun is perfect for garlic.

Harvesting & Storage: Harvest when the leaves turn brown and die down. Shake off loose dirt and cut off stringy rootlets. Let the bulbs dry for a day or two, then braid them. To do this, soak the tops in water for about an hour or until pliable. Braid the leaves tightly together, adding another bunch with each twist, and knot at the top. Hang in the kitchen and remove cloves as needed.

LAVENDER *(Lavendula angustifolia)*

The latin root for lavender is "to wash or bathe". This popular herb is one of the most appreciated, because of its fragrance as well as steady tradition of medicinal uses.

Key Actions: Antispasmodic & carminative, antibacterial & antiseptic, antidepressant & nerve tonic, topical circulatory stimulant.

Cultivation: Prefers alkaline soil in a sunny position. Sow seeds in autumn or take a cutting in summer. Plants soon become woody and need pruning in spring, and, more lightly, after flowering. Some varieties are less hardy and may be damaged by frost.

Harvesting & Storage: Collect stems as the flowers begin in summer and hang to dry in small bunches covered with a loosely tied paper bag. When dry, shake the dried flowers from stems and store away from direct sunlight in a cool, dry place.

LOBELIA *(Lobelia inflata)*

Lobelia has a colorful history and is marked with controversy. Strongly emetic when taken in large doses, but in smaller doses a powerful relaxant and bronchial dilator. It has earned the names "gag root" and "puke weed".

Key Actions: Bronchial dilator, emetic, sedative, antispasmodic, promotes sweating.

Cultivation: Grows best in a rich moist loamy soil. It will tolerate full sun or partial shade. Sow seeds (which can be tricky) or purchase established plants.

Harvesting & Storage: Collect the whole herb while still in flower after a few seed capsule develop. Hang to dry in small bunches. Store in a cool dry place.

MARIGOLD *(Calendula officinalis)*

An effective antiseptic, pot marigold was used in medieval times to counter "plague and pestilence."

Key Actions: Anti-inflammatory, antimicrobial, heals wounds, astringent;

Cultivation: Thrives in full sun and all soils. Sow seeds in spring. Plant greenhouse grown seedlings outside in early summer. Self-seeds. **Caution: Do not confuse with the** **Tagetes species of marigolds.**

Harvest & Storage: Harvest flowerheads in summer. Dry on trays, remove dried petals, and store out of sunlight in a cool, dry place.

MARSHMALLOW *(Althea officinalis)*

Marshmallow has been regarded as a healing herb since ancient Egyptian times. The roots and leaves are extremely mucilaginous, or gluey, and help restore tissues.

Key Actions: Soothing, diuretic, expectorant, heals wounds.

Cultivation: Prefers a sunny site in moist or wet conditions. Sow seeds in late summer or divide the plants in autumn.

Harvesting & Storage: Collect flowers, leaves, and stems in summer and the root from 2 year old (or older) plants in the autumn. Hang to dry in small bunches and then remove the leaves, discarding the thick stem. Dry the flowers separately on trays. Store in a cool, dry place away from direct sunlight.

MILK THISTLE *(Silybum marianum)*

Medieval legend refers to the white mottling of milk thistle leaves being caused by a drop of the Virgin Mary's milk. This liver treating herb is both very effective and very safe.

Key Actions: protects the liver from toxins, both preventative and curative.

Cultivation: Easily grown from seed which germinates readily. Thrives in poor, dry soils. Seeds are sown in early spring or late fall, and germinate in one to two weeks.

Harvesting & Storage: Harvest in the second year. Once seeds are ripe and ready for harvest, they easily shatter from the receptacle, making handling difficult. The seed must be rubbed to remove the plume of papas from its crown.

MINTS *(Mentha species, including peppermint, spearmint)*

There are at least 2,300 variations of mint. Consumed primarily as tea, but full of medicinal benefits.

Key Actions: Antispasmodic, stimulates digestion, soothes nerves.

Cultivation: Begin with stem or root cuttings. Buying and planting seed is a futile effort. Mints require a rich, moist soil with good drainage. You may want to put your mint in a planter box or put barriers below the surface of the ground to keep it from spreading. This hardy plant will take over the whole yard if you don't prevent it.

Harvesting & Storage: Harvest as mint reaches full bloom. Dry the leaves in open air. Once dried the leaves crack from the stem easily and can be stored in plastic bags or a sealed jar.

ROSEMARY *(Rosmarinus officinalis)*

Herbalists have long regarded rosemary as a potent tonic and believed it could "gladden the heart". It is warming and has a stimulating effect on the nervous system.

Key Actions: Tonic & stimulant nervine, circulatory & heart tonic, antibacterial & antiseptic, antidepressant, carminative.

Cultivation: Prefers well-drained, slightly alkaline soil in full sun. Can be grown from seed sown in spring, although it is more usually propagated from cuttings in summer. Remove frost-damaged or straggly shoots in spring and prune after flowering in late spring. Shelter in winter, since cold, wet weather can cause the stems to rot.

Harvesting & Storage: Because it is an evergreen, rosemary can be collected and used fresh throughout the year. For dried stock, collect flowering tops and leaves in spring and hang to dry in bunches. When dry, remove the leaves from the woody stems and store in a cool, dry place.

ST. JOHN'S WORT *(Hypericum perforatum)*

Traditionally regarded as a wound herb, St. John's wort is now recognized as a potent antidepressant. It is widely prescribed by German doctors as an alternative to drugs.

Key Actions: antidepressant & sedative, mild analgesic, anti-inflammatory, antiviral & astringent.

Cultivation: Prefers dry, sunny conditions. Sow seeds or propagate by root division in autumn or spring. Tends to self-seed and become invasive (unruly).

Harvest & Storage: Collect the flowering tops and use fresh or dried to make oils. For infusions or tinctures, gather stems during the flowering period in the summer, hang to dry in small bunches, then crumble leaves and flowers. Store in a cool, dry place away from direct sunlight. Tincturing fresh flowers is best.

THYME *(Thymus vulgaris)*

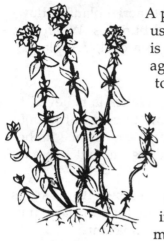

A potent antiseptic, thyme has long been used to treat lung infections. The name is derived from a Greek word for courage, indicating its use as a stimulating tonic.

Key Actions: antiseptic, antimicrobial & antiviral, antispasmodic & carminative, stimulating tonic, expectorant.

Cultivation: Intolerant of wet soil in the winter. Propagate from seed sown in spring, from cuttings taken in summer, or by dividing established plants in late summer. Has tendency to become woody after a couple of years, so prune hard in early spring and clip lightly after flowering to encourage new growth.

Caution: Avoid high doses in pregnancy.

Harvesting & Storage: Collect aerial parts during flowering in summer and hang to dry in small bunches. When dry, crumble leaves and smaller stems and store in clean glass jars in a cool, dark, dry place. Harvest fresh sprigs throughout the growing season.

VERVAIN *(Verbena officinalis)*

Regarded as sacred by both the Romans and Druids, vervain was once believed to have magical properties. Today it is mainly used for nervous disorders and liver problems.

Key Actions: Relaxing & sedative, bile stimulant, uterine stimulant, promotes sweating & milk flow.

Cultivation: Prefers well-drained soil and a sunny position, but is tolerant of partial shade and thrives in poor, chalky soils. Sow seed in spring or autumn or divide established plants in spring. Stem cuttings can be taken in early autumn. Caution: Do not take in pregnancy, although it can be helpful during labor.

Harvesting & Storage: Collect the whole aerial plant as flowering begins and hang to dry in small bunches. When dry, crumble and store in clean, glass jars in a cool, dry place.

YARROW *(Achillea millefolium)*

The Greek hero Achilles is believed to have used yarrow to cure battle injuries in the Trojan War - hence its botanical name and its ancient use as a wound herb.

Key Actions: promotes sweating, stops bleeding, anti-inflammatory, urinary antiseptic, blood vessel relaxant

Cultivation: Prefers hot, dry conditions with well-drained soil. Sow seeds in spring or propagate established plants by root division in spring. Yarrow can take over and self-seeds.

Harvesting & Storage: Gather stems during the flowering period in summer. Hang to dry in small bunches, and then crumble the leaves discarding any thick stems. Store in a cool, dry place away from direct sunlight. Flowers can be gathered separately and dried in trays or on a dehydrator.

Chapter 21

BUILDING YOUR OWN FIRST AID KIT

FIRST AID KITS

Make this handbook a part of your first-aid kit. Assemble your kit now, before you need it. Tailor the contents to fit your family's particular needs and lifestyle. Don't add first-aid supplies to the jumble of toothpaste and cosmetics in the medicine cabinet. Instead, assemble them in a kit such as Western Botanicals' Herbal First Aid kit or a fishing tackle box or small tool chest. Make sure that everything in the kit is labeled clearly. Any bottle or container that is not labeled should be discarded.

Be sure not to lock the box or First-Aid kit. Otherwise you may find yourself hunting for the key when seconds count. An herbal first-aid kit is ideal, because there are no harmful drugs or medicines that could cause poisoning or harm to a child or animal. Check your kit periodically to restock your kit.

Herbal Formulae

1. Immune Boost - used for infectious illness, feverish illness.
2. Colon Cleanse - an excellent herbal laxative that assists with elimination while building tone and strengthening the colon.
3. Colon Detox - used to deeply cleanse the colon, for diarrhea, used as a drawing poultice, for stings and bites.

4. Digestion Aid Formula - for indigestion, upset stomach or gastritis.

5. CTR ointment - used to speed healing of cuts, wounds, abrasions, bruises. Any type of wound healing.

6. Lung Formula - for asthma, pneumonia, bronchitis, any respiratory problem.

7. Deep Heat oil or ointment - for sprains, strains and muscular pain. Also relieves earache pain used in a non ruptured ear.

8. CTR syrup - used internally to speed the healing of any injury where tissue has been disrupted or damaged.

9. Kidney-Bladder Formula - for urinary tract infection, incontinence, general edema (swelling) or kidney and bladder concerns.

10. Liver-Gallbladder Formula - for any liver condition (infectious or toxic), for digestive complaints.

11. Nerve Calm Formula - for nervous tension, irritation, insomnia, panic attacks.

12. Anti-Septic Formula - used primarily to cleanse and disinfect wounds.

13. Herbal Tooth Powder - for any teeth or gum infection or weakness.

14. Herbal Ear drops - used for earaches in the ears as well as around the ears. Used also externally for cysts or swellings.

15. Herbal Mouthwash - for gingivitis, pyorrhea, mouth sores.

16. Female Balance Formula - for any hormonally related female condition.

17. Anti-Plague Syrup - for any infectious condition that can result in death. Used to boost and stimulate the immune system.

Single Herbs

1. Cayenne Tincture - used to stop bleeding, for shock and to increase circulation.

2. Cayenne powder - bleeding, shock and circulation.

3. Lobelia tincture - relaxant, anti-spasmodic, for asthma, an emetic.

4. Peppermint essential oil - for digestion, opens lungs and sinus.

5. Tea Tree oil - topical anti-fungal, anti-bacterial.

6. Clove oil - topical pain reliever for teeth or mouth sores.

7. Lavender oil - topical anti-bacterial, for insect bites.

8. Garlic oil - for ear infections, topical anti-bacterial, anti-fungal.

9. Slippery Elm bark powder - soothes digestive upsets, for colitis.

10. Castor oil - used topically as a fomentation to relieve and reduce pain, inflammation, growths, and swellings.

11. Shepherd's Purse tincture - stops excessive bleeding, especially menstrual.

12. Crystallized Ginger or ginger capsules- used for motion sickness, nausea or digestive complaints.

13. Yarrow Tincture - for fever.

14. Plantain Tincture - for bites, stings, or skin irritations.

15. Mullein Tincture - calms and soothes digestion.

16. Horsetail Tincture - for muscle cramps.

Miscellaneous Products

1. Sea Salt - for mineral replacement in dehydration.

2. Soap - liquid antibacterial or Castile soap - to clean wounds and skin.

3. Epsom Salt - used to draw out toxins and radiation. Used in a bath.

4. Apple Cider Vinegar - for internal arthritis and to wash the skin.

5. Baking Soda - used to neutralize acid burns, for rehydration, insect bites.

6. Miso - used nutritionally to ward off the effects of radiation.

7. Rubbing Alcohol or alcohol preps - used to clean around wounds.

Tools

1. Tweezers - for removal of splinters or debris from skin.
2. Scissors - to cut bandages, cloth, etc.
3. Thermometer - for taking temperatures.
4. Tongue Depressors -used finger splints.
5. Tape - to adhere bandages.
6. Snake Bite kit - in addition to snake bites, use for spider or insect bites. The Extractor™ is a good one to have.
7. Cotton applicator - Q-tips - to apply herbs in small areas or to scrub or clean tissue.
8. Splinter removers - more customized than general tweezers.
9. Ice pack- instant - for sprains, strains, contusions. The I. in R.I.C.E. (rest, ice, compress, elevate).
10. ANA Emergency Insect-Sting Kit - for allergic or anaphylactic emergencies.
11. Otoscope - this tool can be purchased inexpensively to view the ear canal.
12. Stethoscope & Blood Pressure Cuff - to monitor blood pressure and to listen to heart and lungs.
13. Nail clippers - specialized tool for nails (ingrown).
14. Bulb Syringe - to forcefully rinse wounds, for small enemas, to extract mucus. Sterilize after every use.
15. Hot Water Bottle/Enema Bag/Douche.
16. Dental Mirror - to view mouth and teeth.

Bandages

1. 16 - Band-Aids - 1/2" x 3"
2. 16 - Band-Aids - 3/4 " x 4"
3. 16 - Band-Aids - knuckles
4. Ace Bandage 2"
5. Ace Bandage 3"
6. Ace Bandage 6"
7. Flannel - 11" x 14"
8. 3 - gauze - 3"x 8" pad

9. 3 - gauze 2"x2"

10. 2 - gauze 3"x3"

11. 2 - gauze 4"x4"

12. 2 - gauze 2"roll

13. 1 - gauze 3"roll

14. Waterproof tape

15. Vinyl examination gloves - 6 to 10.

16. 2 - Feminine napkins - for any heavy bleeding (not just female concerns).

17. Triangular bandage - for arm sling or ankle wrap.

18. Moleskin - use for blisters.

19. Sam Splint - used for arms, legs, ankle, neck.

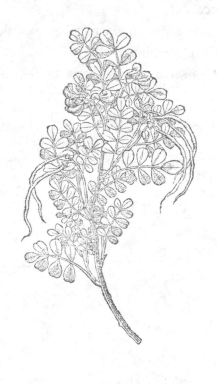

REFERENCES

Herbs & Herbal Products

Western Botanicals, Inc.
7341 Winding Way
Fair Oaks, CA 95628
800-651-4372
www.westernbotanicals.com

Western Botanicals provides:

- Completed herbal remedies (tinctures, syrups, etc.) as described in this book.
- Bulk herbs (by the ounce or the pound).
- Herb Kits – to assist you in making your own remedies at home.
- Herbal First Aid Kits.

Internatural
33719 116th Street
Box HFA
Twin Lakes, WI 53181 USA
800-643-4221 (toll free order line)
262-889-8581 (office phone)
262-889-8591 (fax)
e-mail:
internatural@lotuspress.com
web: www.internatural.com
Retail mail order and internet seller of essential oils, herbs, spices, suppliments, herbal remedies, incense, books and other supplies.

Herb Pharm
347 E. Fork Road
Box 116
Williams, OR

503- 846-7178
For quality tinctures

Blessed Herbs
109 Barre Plains
Oakham, MA 01068
800-489-4372
For bulk herbs

Pacific Botanicals
4350 Fish Hatchery Road
Grant's Pass, OR 9752
503-479-7777
For bulk herbs, dried or fresh

Live Plants & Seeds

Seeds of Change
P.O. Box 15700
Sante Fe, NM 87506-5700
505-438-8080
www.seedsofchange.com

Mountain Valley Growers
38325 Pepperwood Road
Squaw Valley, CA 93675
559-338-2775
www.mountainvalleygrowers.com

Schools

The School of Natural Healing
P.O. Box 412
Springville, UT 84663
800-372-8255
www.schoolofnaturalhealing.com
Herb and natural health care correspondence course work, seminars.

BIBLIOGRAPHY

Balch, James F., Phyllis A. Balch, *Prescription for Nutritional Healing.*

A Barefoot Doctor's Manual; The Official Chinese Paramedical Manual; published in the U.S. 1977.

Berkow, Robert M.D. Editor in Chief. *The Merck Manual of Diagnosis and Therapy.*

Biser, Sam. *Save - your- life Herbal Video Collection.* 1995

Biser, Sam. *When nothing else works...Top Ten Herbs to Cure Big Diseases.* 1998.

Chevallier, Andrew. *The Encyclopedia of Medicinal Plants.*

Chopra, Deepak, M.D., *Journey into Healing: Awakening the Wisdom Within You.* 1994.

Christensen, Kyle, D.C. *Western Botanicals' Health Guide.*

Christopher, John. *School of Natural Healing.* 1976.

Clark, Hulda, PhD., N.D. *The Cure for All Disease.* 1995.

Crawford, Amanda McQuade, M.N.I.M.H., *Herbal Remedies for Women.* 1997.

Forgey, William, M.D. *Wilderness Medicine, Beyond First Aid.*

Foster, Steven. *Herbal Renaissance.* 1984.

Goldberg, Burton. *Alternative Medicines, The Definitive Guide.* 1993.

Goldberg, Burton. *Alternative Medicines Guide; Women's Health Series 1.* 1998.

Hafen, Brent, Keith Karren. *Pre-Hospital Emergency Care & Crisis Intervention.*

Heinerman, John. *First Aid with Herbs, Tried and true health care in emergencies and minor illnesses.* 1983.

Hobbs, Christopher. *Foundations of Health; The Liver & Digestive Herbal.* 1992

Jensen, Bernard. *Food Healing for Man.* 1983.

Kabat-Zinn, Jon. *Wherever you go, there you are.*

King, Kurt, MH. *Herbs to the Rescue, Herbal First Aid Handbook.*

Lane, A.G. Keryn, Editor. *The Merck Manual of Medical Information; Home Edition.*

Levine, Stephen. *Healing into Life and Death.*

Milne, Robert, M.D., Blake More, Burton Goldberg. *An Alternative Medicine Definitive Guide to Headaches.* 1997.

Moore, Michael. Internet; *Herbal Manual, Specific Indications for Herbs in General Use.* 1994.

Nambudripad, Devi S., D.C., *Say Goodbye to Illness.* 1993.

Ody, Penelope. *Herbs for First Aid.* 1997.

Ody, Penelope. *The Complete Medicinal Herbal.*

Schafer, R.C., D.C., F.I.C.C., *Chiropractic Management of Sports and Recreational Injuries.*

Schneider, Richard C., M.D., John C. Kennedy, M.D., F.R.C.S., Marcus L. Plant, J.D., M.A. *Sports Injuries, Mechanisms, Prevention, and Treatment.* Williams & Wilkins Publisher.

Upledger, John, D.O. *CranioSacral Therapy.*

Upledger, John, D.O. *Your Inner Physician and You.*

INDEX

ABOUT THE AUTHOR

DR. KYLE CHRISTENSEN

Dr. Christensen is a practicing chiropractor, master herbalist and naturopathic physician. He is the co-founder of Western Botanicals, an herbal manufacturing company, which specializes in organic herbal remedies. Western Botanicals' products can be found in health food stores and doctors offices across the country. Dr. Christensen's expertise lies in treating a myriad of conditions using herbal cleanses, natural therapies and chiropractic health care. Dr. Christensen has conducted regular herbal workshops around the country striving to have "An Herbalist in Every Home". Dr. Christensen has a practice in Citrus Heights and a rehabilitation facility in Orangevale, California. He has run marathons, participated in century bike rides, triathlons, and was once an avid rock climber. He is passionate about gardening, cooking, wood carving and music (playing piano, guitar, harp, clarinet, various flutes and anything else he can get his hands on). He and his wife, Trish, have 6 children.